PIVOT YOUR WAY TO HEALTH

Reclaim Your Power. Restore Your Confidence.
Lead with purpose. *A Guide for Women.*

Yolanda Moore

Pivot Your Way to Health: Reclaim Your Power. Restore Your Confidence. Lead with Purpose. A Guide for Women

Copyright © 2025 by Yolanda Moore

All rights reserved. No part of this publication may be reproduced, stored in a retrieval system, or transmitted in any form by any means, electronic, mechanical, photocopy, recording, or otherwise, without the prior written permission of the publisher, except as provided by USA copyright law.

No patent liability is assumed with respect to the use of the information contained herein. Although every precaution has been taken in the preparation of this book, the publisher and author assume no responsibility for errors or omissions. Neither is any liability assumed for damages resulting from the use of the information contained herein.

Published by 33 Publishing via Yolanda Moore Global, LLC in the United States of America

April 2025 First Edition

Library of Congress Control Number: Pending

Print ISBN: 979-8-9878169-9-8
E-book ISBN: 979-8-9878169-1-2
Audiobook ISBN: 979-8*9878169-7-4

Cover & Interior Design by 33 Publishing & Design Group

Contents

INTRODUCTION 5

WHEN WINNING FEELS LIKE LOSING 27

YOUR HEALTH IS NOT A SIDE HUSTLE 37

THE PIVOT PRINCIPLES™ 47

STOP SELF-SABOTAGE BEFORE IT STARTS 67

PERSONALITY, PATTERNS, & POWER...OH MY! 81

THE CEO RESET™ 97

MAKE YOUR NEXT MOVE YOUR BEST MOVE 105

DIVINE DISCIPLINE 119

YOUR NEW WAY FORWARD 131

This book is dedicated to the woman who is tired of setting herself on fire to keep everybody else warm

INTRODUCTION

If you are reading this book, then you and I are probably a lot alike. You've checked every box. You've accomplished more in your lifetime than most people can imagine. Yet, you find yourself stuck in this cycle of juggling motherhood, career transitions, relationships, leadership, and the unexpected shifts that come with aging that NOBODY WARNED US ABOUT!

That was me. By the time I turned 25, I had already lived a lifetime.

Two WNBA championships, two children, marriage and divorce, my mom's funeral, and a heart so broken I didn't know how I would survive it. So I did what I'd been taught to do: perform.

Perform at work. Perform at church. Perform for the people counting on me.
Smile, grind, lead, win…. REPEAT.

Twenty-five years later, I found myself still performing. Smiling, grinding, leading, and winning at least on paper it looked like I was winning.

My experience working as a leadership coach and program manager Nike and Amazon, an award-winning head basketball coach who led two different college basketball teams from the bottom of the barrel to conference championships, more degrees than a thermometer looked really good on paper. And if you looked at my social media accounts, I definitely looked like I was winning. Nothing could have been further from the truth.

In real life, I was losing big time. I was diagnosed with pre-diabetes, high blood pressure, and depression due to chronic stress. I was laid off twice in one year, was served with three eviction notices in nine months, and on top of that, I was in full blown menopause and weighed nearly two hundred and fifty pounds, the heaviest I had ever been in my life.

I was getting dressed in the dark because I couldn't stand to see myself. I didn't recognize myself anymore. I hated putting on clothes because I didn't like how I looked in them. I felt myself spiraling emotionally and physically. I was applying to jobs daily only to get one rejection letter after another and that made things even worse.

Despite all of this I still got up every single day and showed up for my kids. I showed up online. I showed up at church. I was still leading but I wasn't well. Everything hurt – my body, mind, and spirit. I was doing everything in my power to hold onto the little bit of faith I had left. I was crying out to God everyday – literally crying the ugly cry. I was uncertain about my future and stressed out about how I was going to take care of these two teenagers of mine.

During this time, I still had people reaching out to me for coaching and speaking engagements. So I was still leading but I just wasn't leading well. My health was suffering, and it started to impact my quality of life. That's when I knew something had to change. I didn't need another workout plan or diet – I needed a mindset shift. I needed transformation.

I realized that my health is not separate from my purpose and if I wanted to show up as the leader God called me to be then I had to stop treating my body like an afterthought. My weight wasn't just a physical issue, it was a spiritual and mental battle.

So, I made the decision to pivot. With faith as my foundation, I applied a new strategy – one that integrated practical application, biblical wisdom, and sustainable habits backed by science. Over the course of eight months, I lost 82 pounds, and not just because I changed how I ate but because I changed how I thought, how I moved, and how I approached my health.

This book is everything I learned along the way. Now, this is NOT a book about how to lose weight. This is NOT a diet book, and you won't find workout plans in it either.

This book is a leadership manual but not the kind that teaches you how to build a brand or climb some corporate ladder. It's the kind that shows you how to transform your mind, reclaim your body, and restore your spirit so you can lead from wholeness instead of hustle.

Because leading while broken will cost you more than any job ever could.

This is the book I wish I had when I was burning out in silence. This is the guide I needed when I thought God was ignoring me.

This is your permission to stop pretending and stop performing so you can lead finally lead from a place of overflow. Your breakthrough begins with your pivot.

Who This Book Is For

This book is for the woman they call the strong one.

The leader. The fixer. The one everybody runs to when things fall apart. You've mastered the art of holding it all together on the outside when you are falling apart on the inside.

But now your body is tired. Your mind is overloaded. Your heart is heavy. And the weight you're carrying isn't just on the scale – it's in your soul.

This book is for you if:

- You have achieved success, but your health paid the price
- You are constantly exhausted, but you feel guilty about slowing down
- You've hit your 40s or 50s and you don't recognize yourself or your body anymore
- You're ready to lead better but you know you need to feel better first

If you are a high achieving woman who knows deep down that God is calling you higher, but your mindset, body, and emotional patterns are holding you back – this book is not only your wakeup call but it's also your way forward.

How to Use This Book

This book is built around the PIVOT Principles™, a five-step process specifically designed to shift your mindset, help you implement sustainable health habits to help elevate your leadership, and increase your faith to trust God for complete transformation in your mind, body, and spirit.

As you go through each chapter, remember, this is not about perfection. It's about progress.
Here's how to make the most of it:

- **Read Through Once.** Let the stories and principles land. Highlight what hits.
- **Engage with the "Time Out".** The action steps at the end help you internalize and personalize the teachings.
- **Write Your Answers.** Don't skip the reflection. This is where change happens.
- **Come Back to It.** This book is your companion guide, especially in the hard seasons.

This book isn't just something you read. You'll be challenged to apply what you learn so you can see real results.

Why I Wrote This Book

I didn't want to be fat. There, I said it. I didn't want to keep squeezing into clothes that didn't fit, gasping for air climbing three flights of stairs to get to my apartment, or wondering who that was behind me making all that noise when I walked.

But more than that, I didn't want to feel how I felt anymore.

I was tired of waking up tired.
Tired of silently panicking about the pre-diabetes and high blood pressure diagnoses
Tired of pretending I was okay when I was running on fumes.

I know there are countless women just like me who struggle with the societal pressures that come with being a woman. Struggling to be see, longing to be appreciated for the value you bring, and battling countless moments of self-doubt.

Like I said earlier, I was doing everything right on paper: Degrees. Championships. Corporate jobs. Coaching awards. Speaking gigs.
I was sick, broken, and burnt out.

I was unemployed and barely scraping by. Then when it seemed there was some light at the end of a seemingly endless dark tunnel, I was offered my dream job as an assistant coach with a WNBA team, only to have them rescind the offer. They offered me another role only to rescind that one too.

This was it. Enough was enough. I cried out to God. I finally surrendered: *"God, if you don't fix this, I won't make it."*

If you know God like I know Him then you know He didn't fix it the way I expected Him to.

He didn't send a check in the mail.
He didn't drop 80 pounds off me overnight.
He gave me something much better: **clarity.**

God told me, *"I don't want you to be sick. I didn't call you to be sick. You can't lead like this."*

That's when I realized this journey wasn't just about my weight. It was about my witness.

How can I lead women to purpose if I'm collapsing under pressure?
How can I coach others toward discipline when I can't discipline myself?
How can I pray for transformation in others and ignore the transformation I need?

This book was born in the wilderness – when everything I thought made me valuable was stripped away. And in that place, God reminded me that my value isn't in what I do. My value is in how I steward what He gave me.

That includes my health.
That includes my story.
That includes you.

I wrote this book to help women, especially black women, release the shame, guilt, and embarrassment of needing and asking for help.

It's ok to say you're not ok. More importantly, it's ok to do something about it.

Leadership Without Wholeness Equals Performance
Leadership With Wholeness Equals Purpose
Yolanda Moore

GOD DOESN'T WANT YOU SICK

When we think about leadership, we often focus on vision, influence, and impact. But what many of us fail to realize is that our health—both physical and mental—is directly tied to our ability to lead effectively.

How can you carry out your God-given purpose if you are weighed down with inflammation, brain fog, high blood pressure, and fatigue.

For years, I compartmentalized my health, treating it as something separate from my leadership, my career, and even my faith. I believed that if I just pushed through, worked harder, and put everyone else first, I would eventually get to a place where I could focus on my own well-being.

But that moment never came. Neglecting my health slowed me down in every area of my life.

What I didn't realize at the time is this:

Your body is the vessel through which you fulfill your assignment. When you are sick, exhausted, or weighed down by unnecessary burdens, you cannot lead with the strength, energy, or clarity that God intended for you.

God has given each of us a unique purpose, calling, and mission. But the enemy will do everything he can to distract, delay, and diminish you—and one of the most effective ways he does this is by attacking your mindset and your health.

- If you are tired all the time, how will you have the energy to fulfill your calling?
- If your body is breaking down, how will you have the strength to serve?
- If your mind is clouded by stress, poor nutrition, or emotional eating, how will you have the clarity to make God-led decisions?

The Weight You Carry Is Not Just Physical

Many of us are carrying unnecessary weight, and I'm not just talking about body weight.

- Mental weight → The stress, anxiety, and overwhelm that drain your energy and joy.
- Emotional weight → The shame, guilt, and unhealthy relationship with food and body image.
- Spiritual weight → The heaviness that comes from not fully surrendering your health to God.

This weight robs us of clarity, confidence, and effectiveness. It keeps us in a cycle of exhaustion and frustration, constantly feeling like we are falling short – both in our personal and professional lives and in the work God has called us to do.

God's Plan For Your Health

Nowhere in the Bible does it say that God wants His people sick, weak, or barely surviving.

In fact, the Word is clear:

"Beloved, I wish above all things that you may prosper and be in health, even as your soul prospers." – 3 John 1:2

God's desire is for you to thrive in every area of your life especially physically.

"Do you not know that your bodies are temples of the Holy Spirit, who is in you, whom you have received from God? You are not your own; you were bought at a price. Therefore honor God with your bodies." – 1 Corinthians 6:19-20

Your health is not just about you. It reflects how you steward what God has given you.

- When you fuel your body with real, nourishing foods, you are honoring God's design.
- When you move your body with purpose and gratitude, you are treating it as a vessel for His work.
- When you renew your mind and break free from self-sabotaging cycles, you are walking in the freedom Christ died for.

This is Your Wake-Up Call

God does not want you sick, tired, or struggling to survive. He wants you vibrant, strong, and equipped to carry out your calling.

This is your wake-up call to stop treating your health as an afterthought.

- Your purpose requires energy.
- Your leadership requires clarity.

- Your future requires you to show up as the best version of yourself.

This isn't about vanity or fitting into a certain size – it's about living in alignment with the abundant life God has for you.

If you've been weighed down with physical, mental, or emotional weight, it's time to PIVOT.

Let's reclaim your health so you can step fully into your purpose.

Because you were not called to just survive. You were called to THRIVE.

5 Ways Sickness Sabotages Your Calling

- **Sickness Steals Your Clarity.** When your brain is inflamed, your gut is off, your hormones are unbalanced, or your sleep is disrupted – you can't think straight. You second-guess yourself. You procrastinate and spiral into decision fatigue. You're not lazy just physiologically compromised.

    Roman's 12:2 tells us to *"be transformed by the renewing of our mind."* But how can your mind be renewed when it's buried under sugar crashes, caffeine dependence, and silent inflammation?

    The enemy doesn't need to destroy you. He just needs to distract you. And if he can cloud your thinking, he can delay your direction.

- **Sickness Weakens Your Witness.** You were created to be salt and light – to model what it means to lead from overflow, not overwhelm. But when your energy is gone, your light dims. When your health suffers. Your presence suffers.

    - You can still show up…but it's dull.
    - You can still speak…but there's no power behind it.
    - You can still lead…but it costs you more than it should.

The world needs to see what wholeness looks like. And that begins with women like you, refusing to lead while depleted.

- **Sickness Fuels Self-Sabotage.** It's hard to walk in confidence when you feel uncomfortable in your own body. It's hard to make wise decisions when you're emotionally and hormonally unstable. So what do we do? We:

    - Overthink
    - Overeat
    - Overspend
    - Overcommit

We say "yes" to everyone else and "no" to ourselves. We numb with food, binge with Netflix, scroll for hours, then wonder why we feel even more drained.

Then the cycle continues.

Sickness keeps you in survival mode. And when you're stuck in survival, *purpose always takes a back seat.*

- **Sickness Disrupts Your Devotion.** You may love God. You may serve faithfully. But when your body is always breaking down, your time with God starts to revolve around praying to feel better, instead of pressing into what God is saying.

    Chronic sickness steals the intimacy of God's presence. You start skipping devotion time because you're too tired. You stop fasting because your cravings rule you. You stop listening to God because your brain feels fried.

    And before you know it, you're still going through the motions...but you're spiritually malnourished.

- **Sickness Compromises Your Capacity.** Let's be honest. You weren't built to lead while sick. When your health is off:

    - You cancel meetings
    - You show up irritable
    - You feel "off" but can't explain why
    - You lead, but you're leaking all over the place

    Leadership requires stamina. It requires mental sharpness. Emotional discipline. Spiritual discernment.

    When your health is constantly under attack, your capacity shrinks. You start operating in a limited version of your potential. And eventually, you settle. You lower the bar. You stop dreaming. You stop building. You start surviving and you call it "God's will".

    Let me remind you of something this:

> *"The thief comes only to kiss, steal, and destroy. I came that you may have life and have it more abundantly."* – John 10:10

Abundant life does NOT include chronic fatigue, emotional chaos, sugar dependence, or sicknesses that you can prevent or reverse.

Abundant life includes healing, restoration, and vitality. It includes you being fully alive, present, and boldly walking out your God-given assignment.

The Leadership Alignment: Purpose. Calling. Leadership.

Let's take this even deeper – because you aren't reading this book just to learn how to be healthier. That's too small of a goal for a fierce purpose driven woman like you. You're here because you sense a shift.

A nudge.
A call.
A responsibility rising that requires your full capacity.

This isn't about the weight. It's about the weight of what you carry. You are a leader and leadership demands alignment.

Because when you're inflamed, distracted, exhausted, or living in survival mode, you can't hear clearly, move strategically, or lead with confidence. When your body is falling apart so is your clarity. And where there's no clarity, your calling gets blurry. That's why we start here with alignment.

Wellness: The Bridge Between Effective Leadership and Optimal Health

For total alignment, you must understand the connection between your purpose, your calling, and your leadership.

- Purpose is your *why* – your identity and reason for being.
- Calling is your *what* – the current assignment on your life.
- Leadership is your *how* – the way you walk out your calling with conviction and consistency.

But none of these can be fully lived out if your body is sick and unwell.

PURPOSE: Why You Exist

"Before I formed you in the womb I knew you, before you were born, I set you apart." – Jeremiah 1:5

Purpose is pre-set by God. It's Not Random. It's Divine.

Your purpose existed before you had a name, before you had a platform, before anyone told you what you "should" be doing with your life.

This is the big picture. The reason you were born. It never changes. Purpose is spiritual. It's anchored in God's design for your life. It's the reason you carry influence.

Purpose is spiritual, foundational, and unchanging. Purpose is tied to your identity, your influence, and your spiritual fingerprint on the world.

It's why your presences shifts rooms. Why you carry a level of authority that people can't explain but they can feel.

But here's the problem.... you can't walk in purpose if you're always walking pain.

When your health is failing, your focus fades. When your focus fades, your purpose gets fizzy.

"We are God's handiwork, created in Christ Jesus to do good works, which God prepared in advance for us to do." – Ephesians 2:10

Your purpose isn't just about what you do – it's who you are. But to become who you were created to be, you must first reclaim your physical, mental, and emotional strength. That's stewardship. That's wellness. That's leadership.

CALLING: What You're Assigned To Do Right Now

"Each person should live as a believer in whatever situation the Lord has assigned to them, just as God has called them." – 1 Corinthians 7:17

Calling is not permanent. It's seasonal and situational. Think about it. You've had many assignments throughout your life. Maybe you've been a mother, a mentor, a builder, a corporate leader, or a business owner. Maybe you're navigating a new assignment right now.

Callings shift. But no matter what God is asking you to do in this current season of your life, one truth remains:

Every calling requires capacity.

You can't build what God called you to build if your health is broken. You can't pour out if you're spiritually dehydrated and physically depleted.

Sickness doesn't just shrink your capacity – it rewires your brain. You become reactive instead of strategic.
Emotional instead of equipped.
You spin instead of executing.

And listen – you don't need more time.
You need more energy.
You need clarity. You need discipline. You need restoration.
That starts with your health.

LEADERSHIP: How You Carry Your Assignment

"Let the greatest among you become as the youngest, and the leader as the one who serves."

– Luke 22:26

Leadership isn't about at title. It's not about being the loudest voice in the room.

Leadership is stewardship. It's how you carry the weight of responsibility with character, wisdom, and peace under pressure. Leadership is your influence.

It's how you show up and respond to challenges. It's how you move people, solve problems, and set the atmosphere.

But here's the hard truth:

If you lead from an unhealthy, anxious, inflamed space...you will leak dysfunction into your leadership. Not because you're weak. But because you're depleted.

You can't pour from a body that's burned out.
You can't' mentor from a mind that's mentally foggy.
You can't model resilience if your nervous systems is on edge and your immune system is always in overdrive.

"Whoever can be trusted with very little can also be trusted with much." – Luke 16:10

It takes character and integrity to lead effectively and with impact. This isn't just about time management, productivity, or performance. This is about trust. God is watching how you manage the body and mind He gave you.

Because leadership starts in secret. It's what you do when no one's watching. It's how you steward your temple, your time, and your thoughts. And if you want to carry more, you must be well enough to handle the weight of more.

Leadership is not positional, it's personal. It's how you carry the responsibility of your calling with wellness as the foundation.

What Is Wellness?

According to the National Academy of Sports Medicine, wellness is: "an active, intentional, and evolving process aimed at achieving one's full potential.

It's not a static state but a dynamic pursuit involving self-awareness and proactive decision-making to foster optimal health.

Wellness is stewardship. It's not just green smoothies, workouts, or a smaller dress size. It's also not a fixed destination. Wellness is you showing up fully aligned – spiritually strong, mentally clear, emotionally grounded, and physically prepared.

The shift is that you're not just stewarding your body. You're stewarding the assignment on your life. God doesn't want you sick because He needs you aligned so you can lead with power from a place of purpose.

Time Out: Reflect & Take Action

Reflection Questions:

- Where in your life have you normalized sickness or burnout as "part of the assignment?"
- Which of the "Five Ways Sickness Sabotages Your Calling" hit the hardest – and why?
- Which of the three – purpose, calling, or leadership – feels most under attack for you right now?

Action Steps:
- Journal this sentence and finish it: *"If I were fully well, I would show up as a leader who….."*

- Pray this prayer aloud:
  "God, I don't want to perform while secretly resenting assignment. Help me steward my

health so I can carry the weight of my calling with joy, clarity, and strength."

- Choose one wellness act this week that honors your leadership capacity:
    - Prioritize Rest
    - Eliminate One Food or Habit That Drains Your Energy
    - Block Time for Silence and Clarity
    - Start moving your body for at least 20-minutes everyay

CHAPTER 1

WHEN WINNING FEELS LIKE LOSING

"You will lose yourself trying to be everything to everyone, and nothing will feel more devastating than realizing that you forgot to be something to yourself."
– Anonymous

We don't talk enough about the cost of being the strong one. We don't talk about how many high-achieving women suffer in silence because they've been conditioned to believe that asking for help = weakness, and that health is a side hobby — not a leadership priority.

We don't talk about how many women eat their emotions, dismiss their body's signals, and hide behind busyness.

We don't talk about how painful it is to wake up and feel like:

- Your body is betraying you
- Your joy is buried under responsibility
- Your power is wrapped in exhaustion

- Your ambition has outpaced your physical capacity

And the cruelest part?

You're still expected to show up like nothing's wrong.

Meet Dionne

Dionne was the woman other women called when their lives were falling apart.

She was the fixer. The solid one. The voice of reason in every room, every crisis, every hard decision.

At 47, she had carved out a seat at the table that most women — especially Black women — weren't even invited to.

She had earned it.
Not because someone gave it to her.
Because she built it.

Brick by brick. Sacrifice by sacrifice.

She grew up the oldest daughter in a single-parent household. She watched her mother grind to survive and quietly made a vow that she'd never live on the edge like that.

So she worked. She excelled. She did the internships, took the extra credit, stayed late, said yes, got the degree, then another, and then another.

She married her college sweetheart. Had a son. Built a strong family and an even stronger résumé.

By her 40s, Dionne was managing a multi-million dollar portfolio, mentoring young women, consulting other departments, and being flown out to keynote leadership summits on "resilience in high-stakes environments."

But the irony of it all is that she was unraveling at the seams and no one could tell. Not even her husband. This is because women like Dionne don't fall apart. They aren't allowed to. They adjust, compartmentalize, and keep the engine running – even when the check engine light has been on for years.

Although she showed up at meetings seemingly energized and ready to take on the world, what no one knew, not her team, not her colleagues, not even her mentees who adored her was that Dionne was holding it all together on caffeine, cortisol, and an unspoken fear that if she slowed down, it would fall apart. Especially her.

Success At The Expense Of Self

There was a particular morning Dionne would later describe as a turning point, even though she didn't realize it at the time.

It was a Wednesday. She had just landed in Dallas to speak at a leadership retreat. The car service picked her up from the airport. She smiled politely, made small talk, and answered a few emails between terminal and hotel.

She had 90 minutes to rest before soundcheck.
She used 88 of those answering emails.

Fifteen minutes before her keynote, she was in the hotel bathroom. Not praying. Not practicing.

But vomiting. Her stomach had been in knots all day — nothing new. She blamed the stress. The travel. The coffee.

She wiped her mouth, dabbed her lip gloss, and walked on stage like nothing happened.

She spoke about the power of capacity and about showing up when things get hard.
She spoke about leading without losing yourself. And she got a standing ovation.

But afterward, alone in her hotel room with the lights off and her shoes still on, Dionne sat on the edge of the bed and whispered into the dark:

"This can't be the reward."

The success. The applause. The emails. The interviews. The salary.

It all felt… hollow.

She had built a life that rewarded her for abandoning herself.

- She hadn't eaten a real meal in two days.
- She hadn't slept through the night in three weeks.
- Her last three physicals had shown elevated blood pressure, high cortisol, and signs of insulin resistance.
- Her OB-GYN had gently suggested she slow down.

She didn't listen. Because slowing down felt like falling behind. And falling behind was never an option.

So she did what she always did, what we women always do – she adjusted, put on a "happy face" and performed but deep down, she knew that this life, the one she had worked so hard to build, no longer fit. At least it didn't fit the version of herself still living in it.

High Performance vs. Whole Health

When Dionne first came to me, she wasn't looking for a health coach which was perfect because that's not what I am.

She wanted to breathe again but not in a shallow rushed kind of way. She wanted to breathe the way you forget to do when your nervous system lives in a constant state of urgency. That I could help her with.

"I don't want to crash," she said. "But I'm not sure I know how to stop." She didn't need another to-do list. What she needed was a strategy and that, I could help her with.

She told me she had been eating in her car, skipping lunch, doom-scrolling late at night, and overcommitting to tasks that made her resentful. She wasn't bingeing — she was numbing.

Every day was a negotiation between brilliance and burnout. She could lead a team of 50 but had nothing left by the time she got home.

Her body was keeping the score.

At first it was just five pounds. Then eight. Then fifteen. Her face looked puffy on Zoom calls. Her joints ached by midafternoon. Her digestion was unpredictable. Her sleep? Shallow. Interrupted. Restless. She had blamed it on hormones. On perimenopause. On stress. And yes — all of those played a role.

Truth is, **her body was not betraying her. It was trying to protect her.**

Science shows that chronic stress raises cortisol, which increases fat storage, disrupts sleep, slows digestion, and weakens the immune system.

According to the American Psychological Association, women in high-stress careers are more prone to inflammation, insulin resistance, and autoimmune symptoms — even if they "look healthy."

Leadership burnout isn't just emotional — it's biological.

Dionne had tried everything from tracking micros, using meal delivery services, a Peloton she hadn't touched in over six months, and supplements she couldn't pronounce. None of it worked
because the issue wasn't her metabolism. It was her **mentality** around what success required.

Yes, she was "high-performing" but she wasn't well. And that's the difference.

**High performance is about output.
Whole health is about alignment.**

- High performance tells you to grind harder.

- Whole health teaches you to listen earlier.
- High performance claps for results.
- Whole health requires you to *count the cost*.

The Leadership Shift

When Dionne came to me, she wanted a plan.

Instead, I gave her a process. I didn't start with food. I started with *clarity*.

I asked her:

"If no one needed anything from you today, who would you be?"

"What's one thing your body has been trying to tell you that you keep ignoring?"

"What would happen if you stopped managing your life like a crisis and started living it like a calling?"

That's when the shift started.

We didn't count macros. Because we are not here to do math. We uncovered patterns. She stopped tracking what she ate and started noticing what was eating her.

She slowed down enough to realize:

- Certain meetings triggered cravings.
- Certain relationships drained her more than deadlines.

- Certain tasks she called "essential" were ego driven.

Her leadership evolved. She stopped over functioning to prove her value. She created margin in her calendar for restoration. She swapped hyper-productivity for intentional presence – with her team, her family, and herself.

Her weight began to release – not because she chased a number, but because her body was no longer living in a state of defense. Her blood pressure stabilized. Her brain fog lifted. She prayed without multitasking. And she finally slept in peace.

The Biblical Truth That Anchored Her Pivot

"Do you not know that your bodies are temples of the Holy Spirit…? You are not your own; you were bought at a price. Therefore honor God with your bodies."
— **1 Corinthians 6:19–20**

Dionne had been managing her body like a liability. This Scripture reminded her — and reminds us — that **your body is not a burden. It's a vessel for purpose.**

Leadership that costs you your health is not stewardship. It's self-neglect dressed up as excellence. And that's not what God called you to.

Before you turn the page, pause. This story isn't just about Dionne – it's a mirror. And if you're being honest, something in your body, your schedule, or your spirit whispered, "that's me." Don't ignore that because that is where the pivot begins.

Time Out: Reflect & Take Action

Reflection Questions:
- In what area of your life have you called survival "strength" when it's really depletion?
- What has your body been saying that you've been too busy to hear?
- How have you allowed your leadership to grow while your health quietly declines?

Action Steps:
- Journal this truth:
  "I've built _____, but now it's time to rebuild _____."
  (Be honest about what you've built for others and what you've neglected in yourself.)

- **Pray this prayer out aloud:**

  "God, I don't want to keep succeeding publicly while suffering privately. Show me where I've ignored Your nudges, missed Your rest, and misused my body as a machine. Help me lead with wisdom, margin, and maturity. Give me strength to release the habits that drain me and embrace the rhythms that restore me. I want to honor You with how I show up – not in my performance but in my stewardship. Amen."

- **Choose one action this week that aligns your leadership with wellness:**
  - Say "no" without overexplaining or apologizing.
  - Turn off notifications after 7 p.m.

- Go on a 20-minute walk with no podcast, no music, no phone – just you and God.
- Schedule time to rest like your life depends on it – because it does.
- Sit down and eat your meals without multitasking.

The Real Reward

Dionne didn't need another title — she had already earned those. What she needed was to reconnect with the woman she'd buried under performance and pressure. Somewhere along the way, in the name of success, she traded presence for productivity... and called it purpose.

But God never asked her to prove herself that way. He was simply waiting for her to come back.

This isn't just her story. It's the invitation tucked inside your own.

You've mastered how to lead others. Now it's time to lead yourself — with strength, with clarity, and with your health in place. Let's build that kind of leadership. From the inside out.

CHAPTER 2

YOUR HEALTH IS NOT A SIDE HUSTLE

"Do you not know that your bodies are temples of the Holy Spirit...? You are not your own; you were bought at a price. Therefore honor God with your bodies."
— 1 Corinthians 6:19–20

Let me ask you something—and I need you to be honest with yourself. Would you ever manage your business the way you manage your body? Would you ignore financial red flags, skip team meetings, stop tracking metrics, or tell your accountant, "Let's just wing it until I feel motivated"?

Of course not. That would be negligent. Reckless. Unsustainable. And yet, that's how many of us have been managing our health:

As an afterthought.
A someday project.
A side hustle.

We pour into our calling. We show up for our teams, our families, our platforms.
We mentor others. Inspire strangers. Pray for breakthrough.

And then we squeeze in a walk if we have time.
We grab whatever's quick.
We tell ourselves "I'll focus on me once everything else settles down."

But let me tell you this from experience: Later almost cost me everything.

Meet Camille

Camille was a powerhouse regional director at a fast-growing nonprofit. She was respected, admired, and always two steps ahead. Her team called her "The Anchor" because she was known for bringing calm to chaos, solutions to crises, and results to every table.

But when she reached out to me, she didn't sound like an anchor. She sounded exhausted.

"I can't keep doing this," she said.
"I'm always delivering. Always fixing. Always showing up. But lately, I've started waking up angry. Before I even brush my teeth, I feel tension in my body and pressure in my chest. I feel like my life is running me instead of the other way around."

She wasn't exaggerating. Camille had been grinding for so long that she didn't know how to function outside of urgency. She led major initiatives and effectively managed high-level donors.

But couldn't remember the last time she drank water that wasn't from a paper cup in a meeting.

She told me she had gained 22 pounds in 18 months. Her knees hurt. Her periods were irregular.
She was anxious all the time, even when things were going well.

And like so many high-achieving women, she had been told:

"Just push through. Get it done. This is the cost of success."

But she had reached her limit. And she needed help not just losing weight — but rebuilding the leader inside the body that was breaking down.

Optimal Health Is A Leadership Trait

If your clarity is gone, your patience is thin, your mind is foggy, and your body is constantly inflamed — how effective are you really?

Camille was still getting the job done.
But the cost was increasing.

Her doctor had warned her about pre-diabetes, and she was taking meds for blood pressure.
She was snapping at her staff and her creativity — the very thing that made her a visionary — had gone flat. This wasn't just about her health. This was about her *leadership capacity* shrinking because her physical health could no longer support her mental and emotional resilience.

The CEO Dilemma: Executing While Exhausted

Leadership Truth:
High-achieving women don't get tired because they're doing too much — they get tired because they've ignored the systems that sustain them.

That includes your nervous system, your metabolism, your hormonal rhythm, and your boundaries.

I was leading. Coaching. Producing. From the outside, I looked like I had it all together — degrees, accolades, a name in basketball and corporate leadership.

But inside? I was unraveling. I was grinding for the next opportunity while silently managing pre-diabetes, high blood pressure, hormonal chaos, and depression.

All while raising teenagers.
All while healing from trauma.
All while putting on a brave face because — "I'm strong," right?

SCIENTIFIC FACT:
Chronic stress activates the hypothalamic-pituitary-adrenal (HPA) axis, keeping your body in a state of fight-or-flight. Cortisol becomes elevated. Your blood sugar destabilizes. Your sleep becomes shallow. And your executive function (aka decision-making) weakens — fast.

"Let everything be done decently and in order." – 1 Corinthians 14:40

I had order everywhere but in me.

My email folders were pristine.
My Zoom calendar was color-coded.
But I couldn't get out of bed some days without praying I'd make it to the bathroom without bursting into tears.

That's when God reminded me — **order begins with stewardship**.

Camille wasn't failing at leadership. She was trying to lead from a compromised foundation.

"To whom much is given, much will be required." – Luke 12:48

We often quote this as motivation — but what if it's also instruction? God didn't just give you a gift. He also gave you a **vessel** to carry that gift. And if your vessel is weak, inflamed, or exhausted, your gift gets compromised — even if you're still showing up.

Stewardship isn't just about your platform. It's about your temple.

According to the *Harvard Business Review*, leaders with high stress and low recovery experience:

- Lower executive function
- Reduced empathy
- Poor decision-making
- Higher inflammation markers

Your health affects your judgment.
Your leadership presence.
Your ability to handle conflict and cast vision.

Once Camille began to understand that **her body was part of her leadership strategy**, she was able to see her symptoms as signals — not failures.

Leading While Out Of Alignment

Camille didn't just wake up one day out of alignment. It happened slowly, quietly, and with good intentions. She skipped lunch to help her team, said yes to one more project, stayed late one more night, canceled one more workout, and ignored one more headache.

That was until her body and her joy slowly started slipping away.

She had all the tools but what she didn't have was *permission* to stop performing and start honoring her limits.

In our first session, I asked her:

"How would your leadership shift if your body actually felt supported?"

"What if being 'the anchor' doesn't mean sinking yourself to keep everyone else afloat?"

Your Body Is Not A Backup Plan

Let me take you back to when I realized that for myself. I had just gone through a second layoff in eight months.

The WNBA assistant coaching job offer I thought was mine? Rescinded. I had no paycheck, no health insurance, a third eviction notice, and two teenagers to care for.

I stood in the bathroom one morning, staring at myself, nearly 250 pounds puffy, inflamed, and exhausted beyond words.

And I heard the Holy Spirit whisper:

"This isn't just weight. This is grief. This is trauma. This is everything you've survived... sitting in your body."

"You are God's workmanship..." – Ephesians 2:10

Trauma doesn't just live in your memories — it lives in your cells.
It creates chronic inflammation, disrupts the gut-brain axis, and reprograms your nervous system to stay in survival mode.

I had been treating my body like a burden for years. But it had carried me through hell and back — three knee surgeries, pregnancies, a championship playing and coaching career, marriage, divorce, a domestic violence incident that nearly took my life, and the deaths of both my parents.

And I'd never once said thank you.

Obedience Is Time-Sensitive

We don't talk about this enough in Christian circles:

There are levels of leadership that require you to be physically strong enough to carry them.

"Let us not grow weary in doing good..." – Galatians 6:9

Yes, that applies spiritually — but also biologically. When your blood sugar is unstable, your hormones are dysregulated, and your energy is depleted, you're not just weary. You're *physiologically incapable* of sustaining the assignment.

And the enemy knows it.
He knows he doesn't have to destroy you.
He just needs to exhaust you.

You can't cast out what you refuse to confront.
You can't rebuke high blood pressure while ignoring sodium.
You can't declare healing over insulin resistance while skipping meals and spiking your glucose.
You can't mistreat your body and expect it to cooperate with your calling.

The Cost Of Delaying Wellness

Every time you delay your wellness, you normalize dysfunction. You teach your instincts to lead from depletion instead of discernment.

Behind the scenes, here's what was happening to me:

- My blood pressure was rising
- My sleep was broken
- I couldn't focus long enough to finish a sentence

- I was missing divine assignments — not because I didn't love God, but because I was too foggy to recognize what He was doing

Delayed wellness leads to reactive leadership.

And reactive leadership *leaks*:

- You snap at people you were called to lead
- You avoid decisions you were anointed to make
- You miss the move of God because your body is in constant crisis

That's why we don't treat our health like a side hustle. Because the Kingdom doesn't need more exhausted leaders. It needs *equipped* ones.

Time Out + Action Steps

Before you turn the page, pause. This chapter isn't just about Camille. Again, it's about you and how you've been leading your body while leading everything else.

Reflection Questions:
- Have I treated my health as optional while expecting peak leadership from myself?
- What leadership decision(s) have I delayed, avoided, or mishandled due to burnout or low energy?
- Where in my routine have I made space for output, but not recovery?

Action Steps:
- **Complete this sentence in your journal:**
  "My body is not in the way of my calling. It's _____."

- **Pray this aloud:**
  God, I repent for treating my health like it's separate from my calling. I no longer want to lead from burnout. I want to lead from wholeness. Give me discipline to rest, courage to say no, and wisdom to protect what You've entrusted to me. Amen."

- **Choose one habit to reset your leadership foundation this week:**
    - Set a hard stop on work hours
    - Block 20 minutes for movement
    - Eat three real meals sitting down
    - Protect your mornings with prayer instead of productivity
    - Drink 6–8 glasses of water before checking your phone

The Real Reward

Unlike Dionne, Camille didn't need a new strategy. She needed to see her body as part of her *leadership strategy*.

Because the truth is, you can't keep showing up fully in your calling while being halfway present in your body.

And God never asked you to destroy your health to prove your worth.

Your health isn't extra. It's essential. It's not a side hustle. It's the **system that sustains your leadership**. Let's stop surviving. And start leading — well.

CHAPTER 3

THE PIVOT PRINCIPLES™

"You don't need more willpower. You need a new way to see."
- **Coach Yolanda Moore**

Before I could change my health, I had to change how I thought about it. Not just mentally—but spiritually, biologically, emotionally.

Because what I was doing wasn't working. Not long-term. I was on the edge of burnout, inflamed, depressed, nearly 240 pounds, and pretending everything was fine. I knew how to perform. I knew how to execute.

But I didn't know how to *rebuild*.

And I couldn't even see that I needed to—because I was filtering everything through an old lens.

That's how the **PIVOT Principles**™ were born.

Not from a textbook. From *desperation*. From the moment I realized:

"This isn't just about weight. This is about stewardship."

And you cannot steward what you resent.
You cannot be trusted to lead what you constantly ignore.
And you cannot change what you still see as broken.

So let's walk through the framework that changed everything for me.

P: Perspective Shift

Let's be real—your body didn't just change.
Your perspective about it did.

And once your mind labels something as broken, it begins collecting evidence to support that label.
So even when you start eating better, drinking water, or showing up at the gym, if the dominant belief is still:

"I'm undisciplined. I always fall off. Nothing ever works for me."

You'll act in agreement with that identity—eventually.
It might not show up right away.
But the moment you're stressed, tired, or emotionally taxed, you'll slide right back into those old grooves.

That's because your brain always wants to be right.
It will look for patterns that match the narrative you've

accepted. This is called confirmation bias—it's not just psychology, it's neurology.

If you've spent years believing that weight loss is impossible for you, or that "this is just how it is after 40," then your brain will filter out any evidence that says otherwise. It will minimize your progress and magnify your setbacks.

That's why the first transformation is always mental.

"Do not conform to the pattern of this world but be transformed by the renewing of your mind."
— Romans 12:2

Renewal doesn't happen by accident.
It's a decision to change your perspective daily—even when your body hasn't caught up yet.
When I was inflamed, tired, and at my heaviest, my problem wasn't just physical.
It was the loop I was stuck in:

- "I used to be strong."
- "How did I let this happen?"
- "I'll start over Monday."

Even when I started making changes, I was still showing up like a woman who didn't trust herself to finish.

So I had to make a decision.

Not just to do better—but to *see* differently.
I started saying things that felt foreign at first:

- "I am a woman who follows through."
- "My body is healing, even if it's slow."
- "Discipline is in me. I've used it everywhere else—I'm using it here too."

It didn't feel true at first.
But every time I acted like it was, my body and brain began to respond.

This is where transformation begins—not in the mirror, but in the mind.

I: Intentional Habits & Implementation

Willpower isn't your problem. It never was.

You've led teams, built families, managed crises, kept people alive.

You are capable of extraordinary discipline—when it's tied to what you value. The issue isn't your ability. It's your system.

Most high-performing women weren't taught to value their health the way they value productivity.
So they treat food like fuel when convenient, sleep like a luxury, and movement like a chore.
Not because they're lazy—but because no one showed them how to prioritize health without guilt.

And so their habits become reactive.
They skip meals because they're in meetings.
They scroll instead of sleeping.

They eat emotionally because it's the only reward they give themselves.

Here's what's really going on:

The brain is wired for automation.
If you repeat a pattern—good or bad—it gets logged as efficient. So if you skip breakfast, crash by 2pm, and snack on sugar to push through, your brain thinks:

"This works. Do it again."

That's not a willpower issue. It's biology.

This is why intentionality matters.
When you pre-decide your meals, your bedtime, your walk breaks, your recovery days—you reduce decision fatigue. And reducing decisions protects your energy for what matters.

"The plans of the diligent lead surely to abundance…"
— Proverbs 21:5

God is not calling you to hustle harder.
He's calling you to steward your time, your body, and your patterns with *intentionality*.

When I stopped reacting and started planning—keeping it simple, sustainable, and sacred—my energy stabilized. Not because I was more "motivated," but because I had removed the friction.

V: Visualize & Speak Life

You will never become what you cannot see.
And you will never sustain what you speak against.

For years, I was praying for transformation while cursing myself in silence.
I would fast, then whisper: "This isn't going to work."
I'd step on the scale and say, "Figures."
I'd look in the mirror and flinch.

I didn't realize that I was reinforcing the very mindset that kept me stuck.

Here's what the research shows:
Your brain can't tell the difference between something vividly imagined and something physically experienced.
That means when you *visualize* yourself walking with confidence, eating with intention, choosing discipline—you're laying down neural pathways that help your brain build that reality.

This isn't about manifestation. It's about preparation.

You're showing your nervous system what safety looks like.
You're training your brain to expect what God already said is possible.

When I began visualizing the woman I was becoming—not the one I had been—I made different decisions.

I stopped eating like I was stressed.
I started moving like I was strong.
I spoke to myself like I was a vessel—not a problem to fix.

God uses vision to initiate transformation.
Before He told Abraham he'd be the father of nations, He showed him the stars.
Before He led Israel to freedom, He gave them a picture of the Promised Land.
And before He asks you to walk in healing, He asks:

"Can these dry bones live?"

Visualizing who you are in Christ—healed, whole, disciplined, free—gives your body something to move toward. Speaking life over yourself gives your mind permission to follow.

O: Overcome Emotional Triggers & Optimize Metabolism

Most of us don't eat because we're hungry.
We eat because we're tired. Or anxious. Or bored.
We eat because we're avoiding something—or trying to feel something.

That's not a lack of discipline. That's a lack of safety.

Your brain is constantly trying to keep you regulated. And when it senses emotional distress—through stress, loneliness, overstimulation—it looks for the quickest relief.
Sugar. Salt. Wine. Scrolling.

This is how emotional eating becomes a cycle—especially for high-achieving women who rarely pause long enough to name what they're actually feeling.

I used to wonder why I could "do great" all day, then unravel at night.

Now I understand:
I wasn't giving myself what I needed—so I looked for it in food.

Here's what was really happening:
My blood sugar was crashing.
My cortisol was spiked.
My body was inflamed and begging for relief.

Food wasn't the issue. My nervous system was on edge. My metabolism was trying to protect me—not punish me. Once I learned how to eat for blood sugar stability, support my hormones, and actually nourish my body, everything shifted. Not just my weight—but my ability to make better decisions when life got hard. That's why this principle matters so much.

You can't overcome emotional triggers without stabilizing your biology.
And you can't optimize your metabolism without addressing how your life is making your body feel.

When your body feels safe, it stops fighting you. It stops holding onto excess weight. It stops craving things that numb you. It begins to heal.

T: Trust God In The Process & Transform From The Inside Out

This is the one most people want to skip.
Because it's not fast.
It's not flashy.
And it forces you to let go of control.

But this is where the *real* work happens.

Transformation is not about intensity.
It's about intimacy—with God, with yourself, with the version of you that you're afraid to become because it requires letting go of everything that used to work.

I didn't want to slow down.
I didn't want to surrender.
I wanted quick results. A big win. An Instagram-worthy comeback.

But God wasn't interested in giving me a new body.
He wanted to give me a new mind. A new rhythm. A new dependence on Him.

And that required trust.

Trust that rest wouldn't make me fall behind.
Trust that healing could be slow and still be real.
Trust that my value was not in how productive or perfect I could be.

Trust that God finishes what He starts—even if it doesn't happen on my timeline.

The hardest part of your health journey won't be the food. It'll be the faith. To believe that your effort matters even when the scale doesn't move. To believe that your body is not the enemy. To believe that what's happening *in* you is more important than what's changing *on* you.

This is how God transforms us—bit by bit, layer by layer, from the inside out.

Time Out: Reflect & Take Action

Before we move forward, take a breath.

You've just walked through the five principles that change everything.
Not because they're magic—but because they're rooted in truth, backed by science, and anchored in God.

These are the pillars that rebuilt me—mentally, physically, emotionally, and spiritually.
And now they're yours.

But before you implement them like another checklist, pause and ask yourself:

Reflection Questions:
- Which principle challenged you the most—and why?
- What false belief about your health, body, or habits are you ready to lay down?
- Where have you been trying to control the outcome instead of trusting the process?

Action Steps:
- **Identify the principle you're weakest in right now.**
  Name it. Circle it. Let that be where you focus this week. You're not doing everything. You're building alignment.
- **Write a "Health Identity Statement."**
  Describe the woman you're becoming through the lens of stewardship, not shame.

Begin with: "I am a woman who honors my health because..."

- **Choose one micro-action from each principle to practice this week:**

    ⇒ **P – Perspective:** Reframe one limiting belief in the moment it shows up
    ⇒ **I – Intentionality:** Pre-plan tomorrow's meals tonight
    ⇒ **V – Vision:** Read your Health Identity Statement aloud each morning
    ⇒ **O – Optimization:** Eat within 90 minutes of waking to stabilize your blood sugar
    ⇒ **T – Trust:** End your day in stillness with no phone, asking God, "What do You want me to notice?"

Prayer To Anchor The PIVOT

"God, I don't want to stay stuck in cycles You've already called me out of. I receive the grace to rebuild—with You at the center. Help me shift my perspective, speak life, and trust You in the process. This time, I'm not chasing a body—I'm becoming who You created me to be. Amen."

Identity Declaration

I am not the same woman I was.
I don't lead from fear. I lead from alignment.
My habits reflect healing.
My body is no longer the battlefield.
It's the vessel.
And I honor it with strength, with truth, and with God at the center of it all.

Now that you've been given the framework, we can get to work.

Next, we're going to walk through the 5 *specific* shifts that PIVOT unlocks—the transformation you'll begin to see when your mindset, metabolism, and habits are aligned with purpose.

Because once the foundation is set, the pivot gets personal.

5 Shifts That Transform Your Health And Restore Your Confidence

By now, you know the principles.
You understand how to shift your perspective.
You've seen the power of intentional habits.
You've started visualizing the woman you're becoming.
You've begun identifying the emotional patterns that sabotage your progress.
And maybe—just maybe—you've stopped white-knuckling and started trusting God to carry you through.

But let's go deeper.

Because understanding the PIVOT Principles is one thing.

Becoming a woman who *lives* them?

That's different.

What you're about to read are the five *core shifts* I see over and over in women who go from survival to strength—mentally, physically, spiritually, and emotionally.

These aren't mindset tricks. They're **identity pivots**—and they will shape how you show up in every room, every role, and every season from this point forward.

Shift #1: From Self-Neglect to Stewardship

You cannot lead well from a body you treat like a burden.

Most of the women I work with didn't realize how deeply they had internalized neglect.
Not because they didn't care.
But because they'd been praised for ignoring themselves.
Because in their world, skipping meals was "dedication."
Powering through exhaustion was "commitment."
Staying up until 2 a.m. working on a deck or planning a conference or managing the family calendar wasn't a red flag—it was normal.

And slowly, that hustle became identity.

Until they hit a wall.

Until the weight gain made them feel foreign in their own body.
Until the hot flashes, brain fog, and mood swings became unmanageable.
Until their prayers started sounding like this:

"God, I love You—but I can't keep living like this."

Stewardship begins when you realize that discipline isn't punishment.
It's protection.

When you stop looking at your body as a fixer-upper or a problem to solve...
And start seeing it as an instrument of leadership, clarity, joy, and spiritual warfare.

"You are not your own. You were bought with a price. Therefore, honor God with your body."

Stewardship doesn't start with a perfect diet.
It starts with the *decision* to honor what God gave you—not someday, but now.

Shift #2: From Hustling to Healing

High performance without recovery isn't success. It's slow self-destruction.

I've coached C-suite executives who haven't had a full night's sleep in years.
Women who are leading global teams but can't remember the last time they ate three meals in a day.

And when I ask them to slow down—when I challenge the grind—do you know what they say?

"If I stop, everything will fall apart."

That's not leadership. That's survival.

Hustle is addictive because it gives you a sense of control.
But healing requires surrender.
And for high-achieving women, that surrender feels threatening—until it sets them free.

You don't need to earn your rest.
You don't need to explain your stillness.
You don't need to work your body into the ground and then beg it to function.

Healing begins when you learn to stop.
To breathe.
To choose foods that nourish instead of numb.
To let go of the need to prove your worth through exhaustion.

And that kind of healing? It's spiritual.

Because only God can teach a woman to rest without guilt. Only God can make peace feel safe when chaos was your norm.

This is the shift from proving to *trusting*.
From constant doing to conscious healing.

Shift #3: From Discipline as Deprivation to Discipline as Devotion

Somewhere along the way, "discipline" became a dirty word. It got twisted into diet culture, restriction, and shame.

But biblical discipline is not punishment—it's power. It's a form of love. It's an act of leadership. And it's one of the greatest gifts you can give to your future self.

When discipline is rooted in devotion, it doesn't feel like striving. It feels like alignment.

You eat well because you want to be clear. You move because your body is a vessel for your voice. You sleep because you have an assignment that requires energy.

Discipline becomes less about saying no to "bad" things... And more about saying yes to what keeps you aligned with purpose.

I remember one of my clients—an attorney and mom of two—who said:

"I've never had a problem being disciplined at work. But I never saw my health as part of the work."

That's the shift. When you stop compartmentalizing discipline and start living it *as worship*.
You show up for your body because you're showing up for the God who entrusted you with it.

Shift #4: From Emotional Reactivity to Embodied Leadership

This one is tough. Because most women don't realize how often they lead from reactivity. Reacting to pressure. Reacting to old wounds. Reacting to expectations, triggers, emails, text messages, hormones, and the hundreds of micro-decisions their nervous system is managing at all times.

That reactivity shows up in:

- Emotional eating
- Snapping at your kids
- Ghosting your coach
- Skipping meals, then bingeing

- Scrolling instead of sleeping
- Crying in the car, then pulling yourself together before anyone sees

Embodied leadership is the opposite. It's when your body and your choices are no longer hijacked by your environment. It's when your nervous system doesn't flinch at every inconvenience. It's when you begin noticing the patterns—and disrupting them with intention.

You feel the craving and ask, "What's really going on here?" You pause instead of perform. You respond instead of react. You become a thermostat—not a thermometer. You lead your body *from the inside out*. And your health becomes the overflow—not the afterthought.

Shift #5: From Control to Trust

This is the most important shift. And the one you'll return to the most. Because as much as we want strategy, what we really need is surrender.

Control says:

- "I have to fix this fast."
- "If the scale doesn't move, it's not working."
- "I'll start over next week."
- "God, why is this taking so long?"

Trust says:

- "I'm being transformed, even when it's not visible yet."
- "I choose consistency over speed."

- "This is a journey, not a test."
- "I trust God's timing—and my daily obedience is the offering."

One of the greatest spiritual disciplines I've learned is that I don't have to see results to walk in righteousness. I just have to show up—*faithfully.*

You don't have to have it all together to be consistent. You just need to keep choosing alignment over anxiety. Stewardship over striving. Peace over pressure.

Transformation doesn't always feel like progress. Sometimes, it feels like pruning. And trust is what keeps you rooted when the harvest hasn't shown up yet.

Time Out: Reflect & Take Action

Reflection Questions:

- What does stewardship look like for me in this season—emotionally, physically, and spiritually?
- Where have I embraced hustle in a place God is inviting me to heal?
- How does my current relationship with discipline reflect (or resist) devotion?

Action Step:

- Choose *one shift* to lean into this week. Just one. Write it down. Pray into it. And let your actions reflect the woman you're becoming—not the one you're trying to escape.

The **PIVOT Principles**™ aren't a checklist. They're a compass. They're about returning to yourself, with God at the center.

And these five shifts? They're your next move.

Not just in health. But in leadership. In motherhood. In business. In life.

CHAPTER 4

STOP SELF-SABOTAGE BEFORE IT STARTS

"Watch and pray so that you will not fall into temptation. The spirit is willing, but the flesh is weak."
— **Matthew 26:41 (NIV)**

Author James Clear says that people don't rise to the level of their goals. Instead, they fall to the level of their systems. This is so true.

There's nothing more frustrating than making progress— only to undo it. To pray with conviction, meal prep with discipline, even lose a few pounds... and then sabotage it all with a pattern you thought you'd left behind.

You start strong on Monday. By Thursday, you're in a drive-thru line wondering what happened.
You promised yourself you'd go to bed early.
Yet somehow, you're doom-scrolling with a snack you weren't even hungry for.

You said you were committed. And you meant it. But something pulled you back. Again. That's self-sabotage. And while it feels like failure, it's usually something far more complicated.

Self-sabotage is not stupidity. It's not laziness. It's not a lack of motivation or spiritual weakness.

Self-sabotage is a survival system. A reflex. A loop. A subconscious response your brain has built to help you cope, control, or escape something deeper.

It's the emotional shortcut your nervous system takes to avoid discomfort. And in high-achieving women, it's sneaky. It doesn't show up like chaos. It shows up like *coping*. Like "just taking a break." Like "starting fresh." Like "being realistic." But if you look closely, it's the same loop.

Meet Rochelle

Rochelle is a university department chair—a tenured academic with multiple degrees, research grants, and a reputation for excellence.

She is articulate, driven, and respected in her field. She is also exhausted. Burned out. And slowly unraveling—physically, emotionally, and spiritually.

She came to me after stepping on the scale and seeing a number she never thought she'd reach.

"I'm sick of starting over," she told me. "I keep getting to week three, and then I fall off."

But Rochelle didn't "fall off" because she lacked discipline. She had discipline in every other area of her life.

What she lacked was awareness of the **cycle** that kept pulling her back into sabotage.

Here's what it looked like in real time:

- She'd meal prep on Sunday. By Wednesday, she was skipping meals between back-to-back meetings.
- She'd end the day so depleted that her "treat" became the only comfort she looked forward to.
- She'd pray for healing… but secretly berate herself in the mirror.
- She'd try to outwork her guilt in the gym, then feel defeated when the scale didn't budge.
- And the moment she felt shame creeping in, she'd say, "I'll just start over Monday."

That's the loop.

And until we name it, it keeps running the show.

Understanding The Behavior Loop

Rochelle's loop didn't start with food. It started with a feeling – usually guilt, frustration, or fatigue. She'd push through a demanding workweek without rest or real nourishment. By Thursday, she'd be emotionally drained, physically depleted, and low on bandwidth. That's when the loop would activate.

At first, it was subtle. A skipped meal. A late-night snack. A quiet voice in her head whispering, *"You've already blown it.*

Just reset next week." And just like that, the cycle reset itself—again.

This is how it works:

Trigger → Belief → Behavior → Reward → Repeat

It's not random. It's not moral failure. It's a system. One your brain created to help you survive a different version of your life—but now it's sabotaging the one you're trying to build.

Let's break down Rochelle's pattern:

Trigger:

A high-stress day. A tight deadline. A confrontation. Hormonal shifts. Emotional fatigue.
Anything that drained her emotionally or physically without a release.

Belief:

"I deserve this."
"I'll never be consistent anyway."
"Food is the only thing I don't have to manage right now."

These weren't conscious thoughts—they were subconscious agreements.
And her nervous system clung to them because they felt *familiar*.

Behavior:

DoorDash.
Late-night grazing.

Skipping breakfast.
Overexercising the next morning to "make up" for it.

Reward:

Temporary comfort.
Numbing.
A few minutes of control in a life that otherwise felt like pressure and performance.

But what followed was predictable:
Guilt. Frustration. Another failed attempt. Another Monday reset.

And the worst part? Rochelle was making real progress. But she couldn't *feel* it—because the loop kept dragging her back into old agreements. We all have loops like this. Some rooted in trauma. Some in culture. Some in conditioning.

The loop is often formed in adolescence or early adulthood and goes unchecked because it "works" for a season. But when you try to grow… heal… take control of your health… the loop becomes a leash.

And unless you name it—you'll keep walking in circles while calling it discipline.

Here's what I asked Rochelle:

"What are you really trying to fix when you sabotage yourself?"
"What fear comes up when things start working?"
"Who told you that consistency has to feel like punishment?"

She couldn't answer right away. Most women can't. Because self-sabotage isn't about the behavior. It's about *what the behavior is protecting you from.*

That protection might be:

- Fear of failure
- Fear of visibility
- Fear of losing control
- Fear of success you don't feel worthy of
- Fear that healing will cost you the coping systems you've depended on

That's why we don't fix self-sabotage by trying harder. We break it by **investigating what it's protecting.** And that's where we go next.

How To Investigate The Assignment

Rochelle didn't come to me confused about what to do. She knew what to eat. She knew how to move. She even knew how to pray. But she didn't know how to *connect her calling to her health*. She didn't realize that the very thing she kept sabotaging was the vessel God wanted to use—not just for her wellbeing, but for the work He'd assigned to her.

We spent the next few sessions peeling back the real reason behind her cycles.
Not just behavior patterns—but **purpose avoidance**.

"I feel like if I really get it together, then something big will be expected of me," she said.
"And I'm scared I won't be enough."

That was it. Her sabotage wasn't about the food. It was about fear—of stepping into what God actually called her to do.

Because here's the truth most people won't say out loud:

Sometimes, it's just easier to manage dysfunction than to confront the weight of your assignment.

When you're tired, bloated, foggy, inflamed, and exhausted, you don't have to lead boldly.
You can hide behind fatigue.
You can stay busy instead of being effective.
You can keep asking God for clarity while ignoring the instructions you've already been given.

But once you heal...
Once your mind clears and your body stabilizes and your strength returns... Now you're *available*. Now you're *responsible*. Now the work begins.

That's why the enemy doesn't just attack your schedule. He attacks your health.

Because a woman who is aligned, fueled, and fully awake is a *threat*. She's not just consistent—she's dangerous. She walks in discernment.
She shows up in authority.
She no longer needs food or busyness or burnout to give her an identity.

She knows who she is.
She knows what season she's in.
And she knows what God is asking her to carry.

That's what I told Rochelle.

"Your health isn't just about energy and clothes that fit. It's about *capacity*—for the assignment God placed on your life."

"If you're constantly drained, how will you discern His voice?" "If you're always foggy, how will you recognize the doors He's opening?" "If you're in a state of physical chaos, how will you steward spiritual clarity?"

She got quiet. Then she said the words that changed everything:

"I think I've been managing my life like a crisis... instead of leading it like a calling." That's the moment her loop broke.

Not overnight. Not perfectly. But decisively. Because when you investigate your assignment, you start making decisions differently.

You don't eat to cope—you eat to show up.
You don't push through burnout—you build systems that protect your assignment. You stop apologizing for resting. You stop using sabotage to delay obedience. And when that happens, your body begins to cooperate with your calling.

Breaking The Loop: How Rochelle Made the Shift

Rochelle didn't change overnight.

She wasn't magically "healed" because she had a breakthrough moment.
She had to walk it out—daily, deliberately, prayerfully.

And it started with a decision:

"I'm no longer managing symptoms. I'm investigating the root."

We began her process with what I call a **pattern interruption.** Not a punishment. Not a strict regimen. Just enough awareness to break autopilot.

First, She Got Curious

Instead of judging herself after every setback, she started asking:

- "What was I feeling before that craving hit?"
- "Who was I talking to before I lost my peace?"
- "What emotion was I trying to suppress with food?"

She didn't answer these questions perfectly. But she stopped running from them. She journaled what I call her *craving cues*—those moments where her first instinct was to check out.

Over time, she saw the pattern. She didn't binge on sugar because she was weak. She binged when she felt invisible. She overcommitted when she felt unqualified. She skipped meals when she felt overwhelmed by expectation. Once she saw it, she could interrupt it.

Next, She Stabilized Her Body

We focused on small physical wins that made her body feel safe again.

- A protein-rich breakfast within 90 minutes of waking.

- Eating every 3–4 hours—before she got ravenous.
- Keeping hydrating snacks and water at her desk.
- Turning off screens one hour before bed to reset her nervous system.

She didn't lose 20 pounds in a month. But her inflammation dropped.
Her cravings softened. Her sleep improved. Her energy started showing up before the coffee did. And that gave her the confidence to take the next step.

Then, She Began Practicing Obedience Over Outcome

Before, Rochelle would only feel "successful" if the scale moved. Now, she started tracking a different metric: *obedience*.

Did I show up with integrity today?
Did I listen to my body instead of overriding it?
Did I fuel my assignment—or just get through the day?

She began replacing self-punishment with self-stewardship. She made rest a non-negotiable.
She learned how to say no without a three-paragraph explanation. She stopped shrinking to stay likable and started leading from overflow.

Her body followed. She lost 26 pounds in four months. Her blood pressure normalized. She had the stamina to teach, lead, and even train for a local 5K. But more than that? She was no longer living on the edge of burnout. She was leading herself the same way she led her team—with clarity, order, and purpose.

Time Out: Reflect & Take Action

This chapter wasn't just about food, fatigue, or falling off again. It was about the deeper reason you keep circling the same mountain. Because you don't need another diet. You need discernment. You need to name the cycle. Investigate the assignment. And stop managing your life like a crisis when God called you to lead it like a calling.

Reflection Questions:
- Where in your life have you mistaken *coping* for *consistency*?
- What emotional loop keeps pulling you back into sabotage, even when things are working?
- How have you been using busyness, food, or fatigue to avoid the weight of your assignment?

Action Steps:
- **Identify your dominant loop.**
  Ask: What's the emotion that triggers my reset cycle? Write down the pattern you usually follow and what it's trying to protect you from.
- **Create your "Obedience Wins" tracker.**
  Instead of chasing a number, track actions that honor your health and leadership:
  → Ate breakfast before 10 a.m.
  → Took a 10-minute walk between meetings
  → Said "no" without guilt
  → Prayed instead of numbing
- **Investigate your current assignment.**
  Ask yourself:
  - "What is God asking me to carry in this season?"
  - "Where is my health out of alignment with that assignment?"

If you're constantly exhausted, it's not because you're weak. It's because you've been operating outside the structure God designed you to sustain. It's your body waving a red flag that something has to change.

Prayer For Breaking The Cycle

"God, I've been repeating patterns I didn't even realize were running my life. I've spoken defeat over my progress. I've avoided rest. I've numbed what You wanted to heal. But today, I surrender the loop. I lay down control, self-punishment, and the belief that sabotage is normal.
Give me eyes to see where I've been avoiding the weight of my assignment. Give me wisdom to break the cycle—and strength to walk in a new one. In You, I am disciplined, devoted, and delivered. Amen."

The Real Reward

Rochelle didn't need another reset. She needed to understand the rhythm of her own resistance.
And when she finally stopped blaming herself and started investigating the patterns, everything shifted.

She began leading herself the way she led everyone else—with intention, structure, and wisdom.
Not through perfection, but through presence. That's the reward of breaking the loop. Not just weight loss. Not just energy.

But the *capacity* to carry what God actually assigned to you—without crashing, quitting, or running back to old cycles. Because you can't steward your calling while secretly avoiding your healing. And you can't move forward until you stop rehearsing what set you back.

This is where sabotage ends. This is where strategy begins. Not from a plan... but from a deeper identity. You've been circling the same mountain long enough. It's time to move.

CHAPTER 5

PERSONALITY, PATTERNS, & POWER...OH MY!

"Through wisdom a house is built, and by understanding it is established; by knowledge the rooms are filled with rare and beautiful treasures."
— Proverbs 24:3–4

By the time you reach a certain level of leadership, you've mastered complexity. You know how to build systems, navigate stakeholders, deliver results. But when it comes to your health? That same clarity often disappears.

Because no one told you that your **health habits mirror your leadership wiring.**
And that disconnect is where many high-achieving women silently unravel.

You're not failing because you're inconsistent.
You're frustrated because you're applying discipline through

systems that were never designed for your decision-making style.

You don't need a new routine. You need a framework that fits how you're built.

In my coaching practice, I use the ADVanced Insights Assessment™ - a tool that combines three dimensions:

1. **DISC** – How you behave and communicate
2. **Motivators** – Why you make decisions
3. **Attributes** – How you process the world around you

Even if you've only taken DISC, you already have a starting point. But here's the insight most personality assessments miss:

Your leadership style doesn't just shape your influence—it determines your self-discipline.
And when you understand that everything changes.

Breaking Down The Four Styles

Please understand that your personality is NOT your identity. But when you learn how you're wired, you stop fighting yourself and start flowing in alignment with who God called you to be.

Now, let's break down the four core styles so you can stop guessing and start leading—and living—with power.

THE DRIVER (High D)

Primary Traits:
Decisive. Fast-moving. Results-oriented. Focused on outcomes over process.

Core Fear:
Losing control or appearing weak.

Sabotage Pattern:
Goes all-in with strict routines or extreme plans—then abandons them when results don't come fast enough. Constantly restarts.

Transformation Strategy:
Shift from speed to sustainability. Use data, performance metrics, and forward momentum as engagement—not identity. Build systems that reward discipline, not perfection.

THE INFLUENCER (High I)

Primary Traits:
Energetic. Optimistic. People-driven. Emotionally expressive. Highly creative.

Core Fear:
Boredom, disconnection, or being rejected.

Sabotage Pattern:
Starts with passion, but lacks follow-through. Easily derailed by emotional shifts or social distraction. Chooses what feels good over what builds strength.

Transformation Strategy:
Create freedom within structure. Use visual tools, affirmations, music, or social workouts. Tie wellness to legacy and personal vision, not short-term emotion.

THE STABILIZER (High S)

Primary Traits:
Loyal. Patient. Supportive. Calm under pressure. Avoids conflict.

Core Fear:
Change, chaos, or letting people down.

Sabotage Pattern:
Puts everyone else first. Abandons her health when others need her. Resists change that feels too disruptive. Struggles to ask for help or create margin.

Transformation Strategy:
Build slow, predictable rhythms. Set non-negotiables around food, rest, and movement. Lean into emotional safety—then stretch gently into new levels of strength.

THE ANALYST (High C)

Primary Traits:
Accurate. Precise. Detail-oriented. Strategically minded.

Core Fear:
Being wrong, getting it wrong, or looking incompetent.

Sabotage Pattern:
Over-researches. Procrastinates. Fears imperfection, so

delays action. Obsesses over metrics, then burns out from rigidity.

Transformation Strategy:
Simplify. Act before it feels perfect. Use structure—but give yourself flexibility. Focus on consistency, not flawlessness. Learn to listen to your body, not just data.

How These Styles Show Up In Your Health

Let's take this further. Because once you know the internal blueprint, you'll stop fighting against yourself—and start creating health habits that support your leadership.

High D – The Driver

She thrives on performance.
Pushes hard in the gym, fasts aggressively, obsesses over the scale.
If results stall, she gets frustrated and either over-corrects or quits.

What she needs:
Goal-focused programs with measurable outcomes. Built-in competition or personal milestones. Accountability that challenges her to slow down without losing momentum.

High I – The Influencer

She's magnetic and expressive.
She loves new starts, new recipes, new wellness trends.
But she struggles to stick to anything if it's not fun.

What she needs:
Group classes. Partner workouts. A health coach who gives her feedback and encouragement. Visual progress tools (charts, sticky notes, affirmation walls).

High S – The Stabilizer

She's the emotional backbone of her team or family. She'll keep the peace but sacrifice her health to do it. She avoids intensity and prefers familiar routines—even if they're not serving her.

What she needs:
Gentle progress. Accountability that feels relational, not aggressive. Scheduled recovery time. Emotional support and gradual changes that allow her to build safety.

High C – The Analyst

She can quote the macros, list the studies, calculate every plan. But she rarely starts—because it's never "ready" enough. And when she does, she's rigid. One slip-up and she unravels.

What she needs:
Structure with grace. Measurable goals with room for adjustment. Permission to start before every variable is optimized. Trust in the process—not just the plan.

Meet Tanya

Tanya is the deputy general counsel at a global media company. Harvard-educated. Highly respected. Ruthlessly efficient.

Her DISC profile? A blend of high C and D.
Sharp. Structured. Results-driven. A perfectionist with power—and she was burning out quietly.

When Tanya came to me, she had just closed a multi-year merger negotiation. The deal was done. Her team celebrated.

And she spent the next 48 hours in bed—head pounding, body bloated, blood pressure climbing.

"I've optimized every part of my professional life," she said. "But my body feels like the collateral damage."

Tanya didn't need another productivity app or intense cleanse.
She needed a new relationship with her body—one that respected her wiring without being ruled by it.

We started small:

- Meals that were planned but flexible
- Workouts that prioritized recovery over results
- A weekly pause where she didn't track anything—she just listened

Her blood pressure dropped. Her inflammation reduced. And her clarity returned.

"I feel powerful and well at the same time. I didn't know that was possible."

Meet Lena

Lena is the Director of Student Services at a top-tier university. She's relational. Steady. Empathetic. The kind of woman who remembers birthdays and stays after meetings to check on the quiet ones.

Her DISC profile? High S/I.
She leads from connection, not control. She carries emotional weight with grace. But it was quietly crushing her.

"I don't need to be skinny," she told me. "I just want to wake up and not feel heavy—in my body or my spirit."

Her routines? Flawless—on paper. Healthy meals planned. Walking shoes by the door.
But one late-night crisis, one early-morning meeting, one "Hey, can you..." text—and it all went out the window. She wasn't inconsistent because she didn't care. She was inconsistent because she cared *too much* about everyone else.
Lena didn't need another plan. She needed permission.

Permission to lead herself first. We started with:

- Walks that were quiet, sacred – not just for steps
- A bedtime she treated like a meeting with God
- A mealtime routine that wasn't rushed or shared – just hers

She didn't lose thirty pounds overnight. She lost the resentment of never feeling cared for. She lost the shame of feeling like she should "just try harder."

And she gained something even better: Peace.

The goal is to make this wiring and make it work *for* you—not against you. Because the real breakthrough doesn't come from knowing your type. It comes from building the kind of system your future self can sustain.

Work With Your Behavior Patterns, Not Against Them

Let's be clear: self-awareness without strategy just turns into self-judgment. You don't need another personality test that tells you what you already know. You need to know how to use what you've learned to make better decisions—in your body, your habits, and your leadership.

Because here's what most women do with self-awareness:

They over-identify with their wiring.

- "I'm just an emotional eater."
- "I'm a perfectionist—I need structure."
- "I've always been the caretaker, so I come last."
- "I need motivation, or I won't follow through."

They label themselves by their patterns. Then those patterns become permission to stay stuck. But that's not self-awareness. That's self-limiting. The goal isn't to excuse dysfunction—it's to decode it. Because once you understand the *why* behind your habits, you can finally choose the *how* that works.

Let's talk about how.

Step 1: Recognize Your Auto-Pilot Patterns

Your body and brain are designed to be efficient.
So whatever you do repeatedly—good or bad—becomes automated.

These "auto-pilot" behaviors are often invisible until you pause long enough to see them.

For example:

- A High D will skip meals, suppress hunger, and justify burnout as "part of the grind."
- A High S will take on extra work, then emotionally eat when no one's watching.
- A High I will start a 21-day challenge, then feel ashamed by day four because it got boring.
- A High C will delay grocery shopping until she's made a spreadsheet of macros, recipes, and budget—but never hit the store.

The behavior isn't random. It's reflex. And until you name it, you can't change it.

Take inventory of your default patterns when you're:

- Overwhelmed
- Exhausted
- Stressed
- Lonely
- Disappointed
- Achieving

Yes, *even when you're winning*. Because celebration without regulation often leads to sabotage.

Step 2: Rewire the Loop

Every behavior loop has a cue, a craving, a response, and a reward.
The loop isn't just physical. It's emotional and behavioral.

Let's say:

- You feel unseen in a meeting (cue)
- You crave comfort or validation
- You grab sugar or scroll your phone for dopamine (response)
- You feel a temporary release (reward)

Then your brain logs it as: **"When I feel unseen, I fix it with sugar or stimulation."**

That's how patterns are formed. But if you don't interrupt the *craving-to-response* connection, you'll keep reaching for the same fix regardless of if it sabotages your long-term goal.

Here's how to disrupt it:

⇒ **Pause the response.**
   Create a moment between emotion and action.
⇒ **Ask: "What am I really hungry for right now?"**
   This question breaks the trance of habit.
⇒ **Choose a new reward.**
   Something that serves your nervous system: a walk, deep breathing, water, journaling, prayer, music, stretching.

Stop trying to overcome the craving. Focus on redirecting it instead.

Step 3: Design Rhythms, Not Routines

Let's redefine consistency. For high-performing, high-achieving women, structure can feel both comforting and oppressive. If it's too rigid, you rebel. If it's too loose, you lose momentum.

The solution isn't another routine—it's rhythm. Routines are external schedules. Rhythms are internal agreements.

A rhythm says:

- "I eat breakfast within two hours of waking."
- "I move my body every morning—whether that's yoga or a walk."
- "I log off at 7 p.m., no matter what's unfinished."

Rhythms protect your *personhood*, not just your productivity. So instead of asking, *"What's the perfect plan?"* Ask, *"What does consistency look like for me—given how I'm wired, what I value, and what I'm carrying?"* And then protect that rhythm like your leadership depends on it—because it does.

Step 4: Shift from Self-Discipline to Self-Stewardship

This is the heart of the Pivot Framework. Self-discipline is important—but for women who've lived under pressure their whole lives, more pressure isn't the answer. You don't need more control. You need more clarity and compassion.

Stewardship asks different questions:

- What is God asking me to carry in this season?
- What do I need to be *well enough* to carry it?

- What needs to shift so I can honor that call without compromising my health?

That's not a motivational pep talk. That's strategic leadership.

The Bottom Line

You were never meant to fight against how you're built. You were meant to lead yourself with wisdom. When you stop judging your wiring and start partnering with it, you stop sabotaging your health and start stewarding it.

That's the real pivot. Not a new meal plan. Not a workout challenge.

A new way of understanding the connection between how you're designed and how you lead yourself—body, mind, and spirit.

Because if you can lead a team, a company, a family, a department...You can lead your health.

And this time, you won't be doing it out of fear. You'll be doing it from clarity. And that's when everything changes.

Time Out: Reflect & Take Action

Reflection Questions:
- Which part of your personality have you misunderstood as a weakness—when it's actually been a clue to how you operate?

- What's one health habit you've judged yourself for that now makes more sense based on how you're wired?
- Are you currently building your wellness strategy around pressure or around how you naturally lead and decide?
- Which of the four DISC profiles (D, I, S, or C) do you most identify with—and how has that shown up in your health routines or resistance?

Action Steps:
- **Audit your default loop.**
  Identify one behavior you want to change. Write out the cue, craving, response, and reward that currently exists. Then decide what new response you will practice this week.
- **Redesign one rhythm.**
  Instead of overhauling your routine, choose one rhythm to commit to daily (example: walking for 10 minutes after lunch, logging off your devices at 8 p.m., drinking 16 oz. of water before coffee).
- **Speak a new agreement.**
  Write a leadership-health alignment statement: "Because I lead with _____, I will support my health by _____."
- **Revisit your wiring with grace.**
  Forgive yourself for trying to force change through pressure. Reflect on this truth: "God does not require me to change how I'm wired. He invites me to steward it with wisdom."

The Real Reward

Tanya led with precision. Lena led with peace. But both of them—like so many high-achieving women—had to learn to lead *themselves*.

That's the real reward of this chapter. Not in knowing your DISC profile or mapping out your stress patterns. The reward is recognizing that **how you lead others will never be more powerful than how you lead yourself.**

And for the first time, you're not trying to change by becoming someone else. You're building wellness around who God actually created you to be. Your leadership has always been in you.
Your wiring isn't the problem. But now, your health strategy finally honors your design.

This is where the pressure lifts. This is where the pattern shifts. This is where clarity replaces shame—and stewardship replaces struggle. Keep going. You're not just changing habits.

You're becoming the kind of woman who can carry purpose *and* wellness—without compromise.

CHAPTER 6

THE CEO RESET™

"She sets about her work vigorously; her arms are strong for her tasks."
— Proverbs 31:17

There's a moment most high-capacity women don't talk about. It's not burnout. It's not failure.
It's the quiet realization that you've built a life that doesn't include you. Your schedule runs. Your team functions. Your family is covered. But you—your energy, your clarity, your peace—are nowhere in the equation. And because you know how to push through, you do. Until you can't.

This chapter isn't about burnout. It's about what happens after the breakdown—when God says,

"You can keep performing... or you can rebuild. Choose."

My Reset Was About Identity, Not Health

I didn't plan to walk away from basketball.

I planned to walk into the next level of it.

When the WNBA assistant coaching offer came through, it felt like confirmation. After years of grinding—college coaching, personal sacrifice, wins earned not given—it finally felt like the door opened. The call came. The contract was coming. I told my family. I told friends. I thanked God.

And then... silence. No contract. No follow-up. Then, rescinded. They offered me another role—as a scout this time. A smaller win. I told myself, *God still made a way.* And then that offer was rescinded too.

No explanation that made sense. No closure. Just rejection. Back-to-back.

What most people didn't know is that I wasn't just grieving the job. I was grieving the version of me that had always believed basketball would be the vehicle.

That role wasn't just a dream. It was the last thread connecting me to the identity I had built since I was a teenager: the competitor. The player. The coach. The champion. The one who pushed through everything and *won anyway.*

So when it was taken—not once, but twice—I didn't just lose an opportunity.
I lost a part of myself.

And ego? It doesn't grieve quietly.

I felt ashamed. Embarrassed. I had told people. People were excited. I had spoken too soon, and I felt like I had to go back and undo my celebration. The silence that followed was deafening.

And then God spoke—not in comfort, but in confrontation:

"You've spent your life identifying with what you do. I want to show you who you are without it." He stripped what I had spent years trying to prove. Not to punish me. But to protect the woman I was becoming.

I Could Have Spiraled, I Surrendered Instead

I was devastated. But I didn't spiral. I could've numbed with food. Checked out emotionally. Let my body go the way my heart felt. But instead, I decided to build what I could control: my health. And not for vanity. I wasn't chasing abs, and I wasn't trying to get a revenge body.

I just needed to feel *grounded* again.

To feel something other than the ache of disappointment. To remind myself that I was still here—and that I didn't need a title to be whole.

In eight months, I lost over 80 pounds. I went from a size 16/18 to a 6. I reversed inflammation. Regained energy. And made peace with a body I'd been ignoring for years while chasing legacy.

But here's what no one tells you: Healing doesn't require the storm to stop. It requires you to walk anyway—with your eyes on the One who calms it. I stopped obsessing over *why* the job didn't happen. And started focusing on *who* God was calling me to serve.

Meet Brianne

Brianne was the kind of leader companies depend on in a crisis. She worked in organizational development for a global healthcare system, managed executive transitions, and built entire leadership pipelines.

She wasn't entry-level. She was the one creating the playbook.

But the version of her people knew—the one who hosted wellness luncheons and coached directors through change—was running on reserve.

Her day started at 5 a.m. and didn't stop until her second glass of wine hit.
Her team would've described her as "present," but her daughter would've used the word "irritable."

Her husband tried to support her, but he could feel the disconnect.

And the truth? She didn't know how to explain it.

Because technically, nothing was wrong. She was respected. Paid well. Secure. But spiritually?
She was exhausted from maintaining an image that no longer matched her internal reality.

The call that broke her didn't come from work.
It came from her doctor. Inflammation. Elevated blood pressure. New onset insulin resistance.
She left the appointment angry.

Not because she didn't see it coming. But because she'd ignored the signs for so long in the name of excellence. And now her body had declared what her spirit had been whispering for years:

"You cannot keep leading like this."

The CEO Reset™ Isn't A Wellness Trend

Let's call this what it is:
A restructuring of what you call leadership—and how your health has been left out of it.

Brianne didn't need a new productivity tool.
She needed to stop outsourcing her wellness to "someday."

So we dismantled the survival system she'd built.

- She turned off her phone at 8 p.m.
- She ate breakfast with protein instead of coffee and adrenaline.
- She created a two-hour, non-negotiable block for deep work—without distraction, without multitasking, without guilt.
- She started walking after dinner—not to burn calories, but to reclaim her body as a safe place to be.

Slowly, her body responded.

The migraines faded.
The brain fog lifted.
The mid-meeting spirals quieted.
The cravings softened.
The clarity returned.

Not because she found more willpower.
Because her body stopped living in defense.

She didn't need to control it. She needed to stop betraying it.

Health Is The Foundation For Purpose

When you're operating from depletion:

- You lead from emotion, not strategy.
- You confuse adrenaline for anointing.
- You miss God's direction—not because you're rebellious, but because your body is too inflamed to perceive clearly.

Let me say this plainly:

You can't obey fully when you're physiologically disoriented. You can't discern clearly if your brain is always on alert. You can't carry your calling if you're surviving your life.

God didn't call you to the work so it could bury you.
He called you *through* the work so He could form you. But He never asked you to do it while neglecting your vessel.

The Real Reset

Brianne didn't leave her job. She left the woman who thought her worth was in how much she could hold. She no longer calls stress "a season." She calls it what it is—a signal.

A signal to stop. To rest. To rebuild. To lead herself.

Because she finally understood: Leading others well starts with leading yourself with wisdom.

Time Out: Reflect & Take Action

Reflection Questions:
- Where in your leadership have you confused high output with true obedience?
- What emotions have you tried to suppress through over-functioning?
- What has your body been signaling that you've ignored?

Action Steps:
- Journal this truth: "I've built _____, but now I will rebuild _____."
- Block one hour this week for restorative strategy: no screens, no noise, no multitasking. Just God, rest, and reflection.
- Replace one false urgency with a system of peace (ex: automated meals, silence before input, calendar boundaries).

Prayer for the Woman Who Leads Hard but Feels Hollow:

"God, I confess I've neglected the vessel You gave me. I've called depletion strength and weariness obedience. Forgive me. Restore me. Show me how to lead with wisdom, rest, and reverence. Teach me how to hear You again. I submit to the reset. In Jesus' name, Amen."

The Real Reward

Your health is not a vanity project. Leadership that costs you your body, your clarity, or your peace isn't holy. It's unsustainable. You don't need to grind harder. You need to govern differently. Because when you steward the woman God called, everything you lead begins to thrive.

You don't have to earn this reset. You just have to receive it.

CHAPTER 7

MAKE YOUR NEXT MOVE YOUR BEST MOVE

"He who began a good work in you will carry it on to completion until the day of Christ Jesus."
— **Philippians 1:6**

There comes a moment when every woman who leads—and carries, and builds, and stewards—has to make a decision:

Will I continue managing my life like a crisis to survive another season? Or will I lead myself with the same clarity, consistency, and courage I expect from others?

This is the chapter where your health journey stops being something you *start and stop*—and becomes the way you steward the rest of your life.

Not with hype. With intention.
Not with guilt. With grace.
Not with perfection. With maturity.

Because the truth is: your next move isn't about motivation. It's about leadership.
And the first woman you must learn to lead—is you.

Lead Yourself With Consistency

There's a myth that consistency requires high energy, perfect motivation, or a breakthrough moment. But real consistency isn't built in emotional highs. It's built in daily decisions.

That means showing up when no one claps. That means choosing the small, unsexy thing that builds capacity long before results. That means treating your own wellness like a boardroom strategy: with systems, not emotion. Leadership taught you how to make tough decisions under pressure. Now you use that same discipline to:

- Meal prep when you'd rather scroll
- Rest without needing to justify it
- Move your body even when it doesn't look like it's changing yet
- Stay faithful to the process even when no one sees it but God

This is what consistency looks like in real life. It's not perfection. It's presence.
It's not willpower. It's wisdom. When you lead yourself well, your health doesn't become another to-do list item. It becomes a leadership advantage—a stabilizing force that undergirds everything else.

And if you ever feel like your discipline is broken, remember this:

You've used it before—in crisis, in achievement, in responsibility. It's in you. You just must point it in the right direction.

Master Midlife With Power, Not Panic

It started subtly.

I'd be in a meeting, mid-sentence, and suddenly forget what I was saying. Not just a little pause—a full mental blackout. The kind that makes you question whether something deeper is wrong. I'd laugh it off, "Whew, menopause brain," but the fear underneath it wasn't funny. I'd coached Division I programs, built departments from scratch, managed staff and students and seasons. But here I was—sitting across from colleagues, nodding and smiling, while my brain felt like it was underwater.

No one prepared me for how leadership would feel while my hormones were changing.

I didn't expect to be waking up at 3:14 a.m. every night, drenched in sweat, anxiety wrapping around my chest like a belt I couldn't unbuckle. I didn't expect the scale to go up even when I was eating "right." I didn't expect my joints to ache, my motivation to flatline, or my moods to shift without warning.

And more than anything—I didn't expect the **shame** that came with all of it.

Because I was supposed to be the strong one. The strategist. The coach. The motivator.

But menopause doesn't care about your résumé. It doesn't ask for permission. It shows up, unannounced, and demands that you become someone new—or suffer trying to stay the same.

And that's when I realized:

Midlife isn't a crisis. It's a recalibration.

Menopause, perimenopause, the hormonal chaos, the fatigue, the fog—it's not punishment. It's *permission.* Permission to slow down. Permission to reevaluate. Permission to stop leading from adrenaline and start leading from alignment.

I stopped asking, *"How do I get back to who I was?"* and started asking,
"God, who are You forming me into now?"

Because the version of me who pushed through everything with grit and caffeine? She wasn't going to make it into the next season. She was burnt out. Aching. Achieving but not aligned.

And I believe that's what God uses menopause for—not to break us down, but to *break us open.*

This is a divine shift.
A release.
A sacred transition into a wiser, slower, stronger, more surrendered way of living and leading.

Yes, your hormones are changing. But so is your perspective. And if you let it—it'll be the most powerful season of leadership you've ever known.

Here's what I wish more women knew:

You're not losing your mind. Your **brain is rewiring.** Estrogen and progesterone—the hormones that once buffered stress, regulated your metabolism, and supported memory—are declining. That's real.
Your cortisol is higher, your insulin response is slower, and your serotonin dips more frequently. This isn't just emotional—it's chemical. Your body is responding to a shift in instruction.

But here's the thing:

God already accounted for this shift in your assignment.

He didn't forget about you in this season. He's *fortifying* you for what's next.

So no—you're not lazy.
You're not broken.
You're not crazy.
You're being invited to lead differently.

In midlife, God invites us to **sustain with wisdom what we used to build with hustle.**
To stop treating rest as a reward and start treating it as a requirement.
To stop outsourcing our worth to work and instead anchor it in *who* we are, not what we do.

I used to lead meetings, teams, and projects while bleeding, bloated, and brain-fogged. Now I lead from discernment. From clarity. From conviction. I speak slower. I move more intentionally. I no longer apologize for needing margin.

Menopause taught me to **renegotiate my rhythms** without guilt.

I no longer lead by force—I lead with peace.

And I had to give myself permission to say things like:

- "I need a moment before we move on."
- "Let's circle back—I'm managing some mental fog today."
- "I'm shifting my hours to protect my sleep and energy."
- "I'm no longer available for urgency. I prioritize clarity."

That's not weakness. That's *elevated leadership.*

Because the truth is, midlife is the season where wisdom replaces urgency.
Where discernment replaces grind.
Where boundaries become sacred.
And where your voice finally starts to match your vision.

You don't have to panic when your body changes.

You don't have to hide under Spanx and shame and pretend it's not happening.

You get to *pivot.*
To nourish your body with what supports you.
To move in ways that feel like strength instead of punishment. To speak up about what you need.
To own your seat at the table without performing for it.

You get to lead.
Fully. Powerfully. In purpose.

Not despite menopause—but *because* of what it's revealing in you.

Here's what's really happening in your body:

- **Estrogen** is declining—this impacts brain function, bone density, mood, and your ability to metabolize carbs efficiently. It's why your sleep suffers and weight shifts to your midsection.
- **Progesterone** is dropping—leading to irritability, anxiety, and disrupted sleep. This hormone used to "calm" your system.
- **Insulin sensitivity** is changing—your body doesn't handle sugar and carbs the way it used to, which can create or worsen insulin resistance.
- **Cortisol is more reactive**—your body becomes more sensitive to stress, meaning what didn't bother you before now feels overwhelming.

It's not just a hormone issue. It's a leadership reset.

Because your body is sending you new data. And as a leader, your job is to listen, adapt, and align—not ignore, push, and perform.

So how do you lead well in this season?

Meet Adrienne

Adrienne didn't look like she was falling apart.

She was polished. Professional. Poised. The kind of woman who always had a charger, an extra pair of flats in her bag, and a perfectly timed answer in high-stakes meetings.

At 53, she'd spent over two decades climbing the ladder in corporate marketing—navigating layoffs, industry shifts, and the unspoken complexities of being the only Black woman in most rooms.

She had earned her seat at the table. But somewhere along the way, she'd stopped feeling like she belonged in her own body.

When Adrienne reached out to me, she didn't start by talking about hot flashes or fatigue. She started by saying, "I feel like I'm disappearing."

She had missed three promotions in the last five years—not because she lacked skill or credibility, but because her performance had started to wobble. Subtly at first, then louder.

She'd always been sharp, creative, the go-to strategist for brand turnarounds. But now?

She couldn't focus in back-to-back meetings. Her thoughts felt foggy. She was exhausted by 2 p.m., wired at night, and snapping at people she loved for no reason she could explain.

She was forgetting names. Losing her train of thought mid-sentence. Reading emails three times before they made sense. Her sleep was wrecked. Her confidence even more so.

And the worst part? No one knew.

Because Adrienne didn't show weakness. Ever. She wore structure, mascara, and a professional smile like armor. But she was coming apart on the inside. And not even her husband knew how to help her.

The Moment Of Interruption

It wasn't a doctor that told her something was wrong. It was a moment in a meeting.

She was giving a strategy presentation to a VP who'd flown in from headquarters. She'd prepped. She had her notes. But halfway through her pitch, her mind went blank.

Completely blank. She froze for six seconds—an eternity in a boardroom.

She recovered. Sort of. But she walked out of that room and didn't go back to her desk.

She got in her car, drove home, and sat in her driveway crying.

That night, she Googled two things: "brain fog" and "over 50." That led her down the rabbit hole of perimenopause. For the first time in her career, Adrienne admitted to herself:

"This isn't just stress. My body is changing. And I don't know what to do." That's when she found me.

The Rebuild

Adrienne didn't need another productivity tool. She needed someone to help her listen to what her body was trying to say.

In our first session, I told her something she hadn't heard from her doctor, her therapist, or her HR rep:

"You're not falling apart. You're being recalibrated and you need a new playbook for this season." So we got to work. We didn't start with supplements. We started with understanding.

She learned that declining estrogen affects neurotransmitters like serotonin, which directly impact focus and mood.

She learned that spiking cortisol (from constant stress and caffeine) was keeping her in a wired-but-tired loop—and that weight gain around her belly wasn't laziness. It was her body in defense mode.

We rewrote her leadership rhythm:

- **Mornings:** She started with protein and prayer—not caffeine and cortisol.
- **Midday:** She created a 20-minute walk-and-reflect block after her hardest meeting.
- **Evenings:** She turned off screens at 8 p.m. and journaled one thing her body did *right* each day.

We also addressed her identity.

She wasn't just navigating menopause. She was grieving a version of herself that had been praised for her sharpness, her poise, her speed.

And now, she had to learn how to lead from stillness. From honesty. From grace.

The Transformation

Three months in, Adrienne said something I'll never forget:

"I don't feel like I'm disappearing anymore. I feel like I'm finally becoming someone who doesn't need to prove anything."

Her sleep improved. Her mental clarity sharpened. Her confidence returned—not because her hormones were perfect, but because she stopped fighting her body and started honoring it.

She was no longer performing wellness to stay relevant. She was embodying leadership that didn't require her to hide. She led a new product launch that quarter—and nailed it. But what she celebrated most wasn't the win at work.

It was the night her daughter looked at her and said, "You're smiling again, Mom."

If you are like Adrienne struggling to lead in the midst of your midlife shift, then follow then do what she did. Anchor yourself in what I call the **Four Pillars of Midlife Leadership:**

1. **Metabolic Reset** – Nourish your body for *this* season. Focus on protein, fiber, hydration, and blood sugar balance. What worked at 30 doesn't serve you at 45.
2. **Nervous System Regulation** – Breathe. Sleep. Stretch. Walk. Rest. Train your body to feel *safe* again so it can stop fighting you.
3. **Mindset Mastery** – Release shame. Reframe success. Rewire your language. You are not failing—you are *forging a new standard.*
4. **Spiritual Alignment** – Reconnect with God's rhythm. Hear from Him daily. Ask what He is *developing* in you, not just what He wants you to do.

Because you're not just leading teams, families, or businesses—you're leading *yourself* through a divine hormonal, emotional, and spiritual transition.

You deserve strategy. You deserve support. You deserve space to evolve. This is not the end. This is a beginning.

Time Out: Reflect & Take Action

Reflection Questions:
- What am I pretending not to notice in my health, my habits, or my spirit?
- Where have I confused performance with purpose?
- What do I need to release in order to become the woman God designed me to be?

Action Steps:
- **Write a Letter to Your Future Self.** Not the woman you're hustling to become—but the one you're finally

giving permission to emerge. Describe how she leads, what she prioritizes, and how she treats her body.
- **Rebuild One Habit.** Choose one small rhythm that reflects the woman you're becoming—daily movement, a protein-rich breakfast, screen-free sleep prep, or 10 minutes in Scripture. Keep it simple. Keep it sacred.
- **Ask God for Strategy.** Set aside 15 minutes this week with no noise, no notes, no pressure. Just you and God. Ask: "What's the next small move that honors the woman You created me to be?"
- **Choose a Health Anchor.** Declare one new standard you will protect this season. (Ex: "I don't sacrifice my rest for approval." "I don't skip meals to keep pace." "I don't lead others from depletion.")

The Real Reward

Becoming the woman God designed you to be is not a glow-up. It's a calling.

It's not about finally being perfect—it's about being *present*. Fully in your body. Fully in your assignment. Fully submitted to His process.

You don't need another plan. You need to remember who you are.
You've already led others. You've already delivered results. Now it's time to lead yourself—with courage, conviction, and consistency.

That is the pivot.
That is the power.

And that is how you make your next move—your best move.

CHAPTER 8

DIVINE DISCIPLINE

"No discipline seems pleasant at the time, but painful. Later on, however, it produces a harvest of righteousness and peace for those who have been trained by it."
— Hebrews 12:11

Discipline is not the absence of desire. It's the maturity to choose obedience even when desire fades. If you've made it this far, it means you're not here for quick tips or cosmetic fixes. You're here because deep down, you're tired of cycling through false starts and breakdowns masked as "resets."

You want the real thing. You want transformation that sticks. You want a life that feels like alignment, not adrenaline. You want to move through your day with clarity and spiritual authority—not caffeine and cortisol. That kind of life doesn't come from temporary motivation.
It comes from *Divine Discipline.* Not the kind the world taught you—hustle, shame, extremes, punishment. But the kind God develops in women who are ready to walk in their next season with clarity, consistency, and conviction.

This is about stewarding your energy—not just your image. It's about reclaiming your power so you can lead without secretly unraveling.

Reclaiming Your Power

Let's talk about power for a moment—real power. Power isn't in how fast you move.
It's in your ability to stay grounded when everything around you speeds up.

Power isn't about control. It's about authority—authority over your emotions, your responses, your rhythms. And that kind of power is not self-generated. It's Spirit-led. It's disciplined. It's discerned. When you lead from Divine Discipline, you don't wake up and wing it.
You wake up and *walk in it*. You show up with structure—not for control, but for clarity.
You pray before panic sets in. You prioritize your body—not for applause, but for assignment.

Because the truth is, some of what you've been calling "overwhelm" is just the result of living without spiritual order.

You're not tired because you're weak. You're tired because your habits are out of sync with your purpose. Divine discipline brings your habits, your hormones, your health, and your headspace back under the leadership of Christ—not culture.

Lead Your Health With Purpose

You are not the average woman. You lead people.
You influence outcomes. You carry vision.

But what most high-achieving women forget is this:

You cannot carry vision long-term in a body that's always running on empty.

That's why Divine Discipline matters. Because when your body is cared for, your brain works better. When your brain works better, your decision-making sharpens. And when your decisions are sound, your leadership becomes unshakable.

That's why I tell women:
Good sleep is not a luxury.
It's a leadership strategy.

A regulated nervous system is a competitive advantage. Balanced blood sugar makes you a better communicator, a calmer mother, and a more discerning executive. This isn't about fitting in jeans. It's about not missing God's voice because you're foggy, inflamed, distracted, and always one decision away from burnout.

What does it truly cost to carry EVERYTHING?

Meet Monica

Monica didn't need more willpower. She needed a rescue from the version of herself she had outgrown. She was 41, a full-time entrepreneur and single mom of two. A powerhouse branding consultant known for helping women scale their online businesses into six and seven figures.

She had the receipts—clients featured in Essence, Forbes, BET. Her work was brilliant. Her voice was magnetic. Her life? On the edge of burnout. When she came to me, Monica was post-launch. The kind of launch people write eBooks about—$32,000 in revenue in 10 days.

But instead of celebrating, she found herself sobbing on her bathroom floor, holding her chest, convinced she was having a heart attack. It wasn't her heart. It was her nervous system. And it was sounding the alarm she'd been ignoring for years.

She told me, "I've built a brand that's changing lives, but it's being carried by a woman who feels like she's drowning." Her hair was thinning. Her cravings were erratic. She hadn't slept a full night in six months. She was skipping meals until 3:00 p.m. and binging protein bars and caffeine until midnight.

Her weight had crept up. Her inflammation was high. Her mood was unstable. And still—she kept showing up online, smiling, coaching, performing.

Because that's what she had been taught:
Deliver the result.
Push through.
Be excellent—even if you're exhausted.

What she didn't realize yet was that her business wasn't her biggest assignment in this season. Her body was.

What You Didn't See On The Highlight Reel

Monica had always been high-functioning.
She grew up the fixer in a household of chaos—the responsible one, the "mama's helper," the one who got it done.

By 30, she had launched her first business. By 35, she was making more money in a month than most of her family made in a year.

But the wiring that helped her survive trauma was the same wiring that made her health feel like a background detail. She didn't just have a fast-paced schedule. She had a nervous system trained to believe that slowing down was unsafe.

And every time her body whispered, "Rest,"
Her trauma shouted back, "You'll fall behind." When Monica came to me, she was not weak.

She was weary. Not just from the business. But from decades of managing everything for everyone and being applauded for her ability to perform while unraveling.

The Real Reset

Monica didn't need another wellness trend.
She needed a new leadership strategy—one where she was the one being led.

We started by reframing her entire concept of discipline. She had equated discipline with restriction.
I taught her to see it as protection.

She had treated her body like an afterthought.
I helped her see it as her first place of stewardship.

She wasn't eating because she was lazy.
She was skipping meals because her brain had been trained to normalize neglect.

Here's what we rebuilt together:

- **Mornings:** She started the day in silence—10 minutes of Scripture, a protein-rich meal, and no phone. Instead of reaching for Instagram analytics, she reached for God's peace.
- **Midday:** She blocked off lunch and ate seated, no laptop, no multitasking. She hydrated like her clarity depended on it because it did.
- **Evenings:** She implemented "shut down" hours: 8:30 p.m. screens off, journal open.
  Not to check off boxes, but to regulate her nervous system and reconnect with the woman behind the business.

And every day, she declared:

"I'm not building from burnout. I'm building from overflow. My health is part of my leadership—not a side hobby."

The Breakthrough

Three weeks in, Monica noticed her cravings decreasing. Her bloating went down. She was sleeping. Not perfectly, but deeply—for the first time in years.

By the second month, her period regulated. Her blood sugar stabilized. She was less reactive. Her mind was sharper in sales calls. And for the first time in years, she started turning down clients—not because she couldn't serve them, but because she no longer had anything to prove.

But the biggest shift wasn't physical. It was spiritual.

She said, "I didn't know how much I had made performance my identity until God stripped my ability to perform."

"I was chasing the numbers but losing myself in the process. This reset didn't just get me back in my body. It got me back in His will."

That's what Divine Discipline does.

It doesn't just give you better habits. It reorders your heart. It silences the hustle. It teaches you how to lead yourself the way God has always designed:
With rhythm. With rest. With reverence.

Discipline: A Divine Leadership Strategy

Let me say this plainly:

- A regulated nervous system is a competitive advantage.
- Balanced blood sugar is a leadership tool.
- Sleep is an asset—not a luxury.
- Clear thinking doesn't start with your planner—it starts in your gut.

- A woman who leads herself well becomes unstoppable—not because she does more, but because she needs less noise to discern God's voice.

This is what I've learned—not just through coaching women, but through my own crucible.

I had to learn the difference between hustle and harvest.

After years of chasing opportunity, the WNBA called me back. The job I had dreamed of—assistant coach. Offered. I told my family. My friends. My circle celebrated.

Then the offer was rescinded. No explanation. No backup plan. Just silence.

Then they offered me a second position. I thought it was redemption. It was a test. That one got pulled, too. And in that moment, God stripped away everything I had attached my identity to—title, industry, recognition. And all I had left was Him. And a body that I barely recognized.

That was the pivot. That was the discipline. Not a workout plan. Not a green smoothie. The decision to *obey* when it hurt. To *trust* when it didn't make sense. To *show up* for my health—not because I felt strong, but because I believed I was still called. And in 8 months, I lost over 80 pounds.

But I gained something far greater: Authority. Clarity. Peace. I didn't just lead a pivot. I *became* one.

Monica's Rebuild

Monica wasn't just a story. She was a symbol—for every woman running a business while her body is screaming for a reset. What we did wasn't magic. It was discipline. The kind that comes from wisdom. The kind that builds capacity—not chaos.

The kind that says: "I don't have to be everything to everyone. I must be obedient to what God is asking me to carry—today." This chapter isn't about grinding harder. It's about *governing better.*

A Final Word On Divine Discipline

God never asked you to be superwoman. He called you to be a *steward.*

That means you:

- Show up when it's not glamorous.
- Eat to think clearly, not just shrink visibly.
- Move because you've been assigned to go places—not to punish your past.
- Rest because you trust that what He's doing through you doesn't require self-destruction.

You want to lead at the next level? Start with the discipline to stop hiding from the body that carries your brilliance. You want to fulfill your calling? Honor the vessel. You want to hear God clearly in this season? Clear the clutter—in your habits, in your health, and in your head.

Time Out: Reflect & Take Action

Reflection Questions:
- What version of discipline have I internalized—fear-based or Spirit-led?
- Where have I been asking God for clarity, but refusing to care for the vessel He's using?
- What is my health saying about how I manage my assignment?

Action Steps:
- **Journal this truth:**
  "I do not need to earn rest, peace, or health. I am already called. I choose discipline not to prove something—but to prepare for what's next."
- **Identify one daily decision** where discipline can replace depletion:
  → Go to bed on time
  → Start the day with prayer + protein
  → Replace stress-snacking with stillness
  → Block time for movement like it's a meeting with God
- **Pray aloud:**
  "Lord, train me to lead myself from faith. I surrender the habits that have kept me busy but broken. Strengthen me to steward my energy with wisdom. I don't just want change. I want to become a woman who walks in discipline, peace, and purpose. Amen."

The Real Reward

You thought the reward would be more energy, better sleep, clearer skin, or a smaller waist.

But the real reward? It's *you*.

Showing up fully. Thinking clearly. Hearing God's voice without interference. Making decisions from wisdom – not adrenaline. Becoming the woman you promised yourself you'd be – before the world convinced you that being strong meant being stretched thin.

Discipline is not what you do to prove you're worthy. It's what you choose when you remember you already are. You've pivoted. Now walk in it – with discipline that reflects your destiny.

CHAPTER 9

YOUR NEW WAY FORWARD

"Now finish the work, so that your eager willingness to do it may be matched by your completion of it."
— 2 Corinthians 8:11

You've read the words. You've reflected, journaled, and wrestled. You've faced the mirror. The memories. The myths. And now comes the moment that separates *knowing* from *becoming*. You were never called to lead from depletion. You were called to lead from overflow.

Because at some point, every woman who leads has to make a decision:

Am I going to keep managing dysfunction?
Or am I going to take back the authority I gave away?

This is your moment to choose.

Optimal Health *IS* Your Superpower!

We've made it very clear by now that this was never really about weight loss.

This was about *capacity*. Because when your body is inflamed, your mind is foggy. When your blood sugar crashes, so does your discernment.

When you are under-nourished and overbooked, you may still get things done, but you're not leading from *wholeness*. You're leading from hustle. And eventually, hustle runs out.

Taking control of your health is not a vanity project.
It's a leadership strategy. It's a spiritual assignment.
It's a sign of maturity and authority. Because you can't carry kingdom vision in a body that's always in survival mode.

You Can't Keep Leading From Empty

Too many brilliant, high-achieving women are walking around spiritually sharp—but physically shut down.

You're managing ministries, meetings, brands, households. But your body is sending signals—fatigue, cravings, irregular cycles, insomnia, anxiety—and you've ignored them in the name of "purpose."

Let me say this with love:

God didn't call you to burn out in His name.
He called you to *build* from overflow.

Leadership that depletes your temple is not stewardship.
It's disobedience with a spiritual label.

And now you know better.
Now you *see* it.

So now... you lead differently.

The Pivot Isn't About Your Body... It's About Your Mindset

Let's return to the framework that changed everything:

- **P** – You shifted your *Perspective* and told yourself the truth.
- **I** – You built *Intentional Habits* rooted in identity, not insecurity.
- **V** – You learned to *Visualize & Speak Life*, not just rehearse failure.
- **O** – You took *Ownership* of your patterns, your process, and your potential.
- **T** – You learned how to *Trust God in the transformation*, not just beg Him for one.

That's not a health plan. That's a leadership framework. And now, it's yours. Not just for a season. But for life.

From Stuck To Strategy

This is your new way forward – not because you're starting over, but because **you're starting from NOW.**

Let me ask you:

- What would change if you believed that your *health* was the gateway to your *calling*?

- What clarity would return if your body was no longer in fight-or-flight?
- What kind of legacy could you build if you stopped leading from depletion and started leading from divine discipline?

You don't need another quick fix.
You don't need a "start over Monday."

You need to *walk it out*—one decision at a time.
Until discipline becomes identity.

The "Healthy Leadership" Recap

As a woman who leads, you don't just need inspiration—you need **integration**. You process life through more than emotion. You process through **impact**, **systems**, and the ripple effects of your choices. You know that your health isn't separate from your leadership—it *fuels it*.

This Leadership Insights Recap is designed to give you a clear, executive-level distillation of what you've just walked through in this book. Each chapter summary includes:

- A **leadership principle** to challenge and refine how you show up
- A **biblical truth** to anchor your journey in spiritual stewardship
- A **science-based insight** to ground your decisions in proven strategy

Whether you're revisiting the book, teaching it to your team, or designing a new rhythm for your own life—this section exists to remind you:

Your body is not a side note.
Your well-being is not optional.
Your leadership begins with how you lead yourself.

Use this as your compass.
Come back to it as often as you need.

Because the next level of your influence depends on how well you **protect the vessel that carries the vision**.

Chapter 1: When Winning Feels Like Losing

Leadership Insight:
Performance without restoration will eventually lead to collapse. You can't serve others with excellence while silently suffering. Health is not a luxury for leaders—it's a leadership necessity.

Faith Recap:
God calls us to lead with wisdom and strength, not burnout (Isaiah 40:29–31; 1 Corinthians 3:16–17).

Science Recap:
Chronic emotional stress disrupts hormones, increases cortisol, and leads to inflammation and energy depletion, impairing clarity and resilience.

Chapter 2: Your Health Isn't A Side Hustle

Leadership Insight:
If you treat your health like a back-burner task, you'll lead from burnout, not brilliance. You are the asset. The more you neglect the vessel, the more your leadership suffers. You can't scale success on a broken foundation.

Faith Recap:
Stewardship includes the body. Rest and rhythm are biblical principles (Genesis 2:2–3; 1 Corinthians 6:19).

Science Recap:
Elevated cortisol from chronic stress leads to metabolic breakdown and poor decision-making under pressure. Executive function decreases as physical depletion increases.

Chapter 3: The PIVOT Principles™

Leadership Insight:
Foundational frameworks build sustainable leadership. Without clarity, intentionality, vision, ownership, and trust, your leadership is fragmented and reactive.

Faith Recap:
Romans 12:2 anchors transformation through the renewing of the mind. Proverbs 4:7 reminds us: "Wisdom is the principal thing."

Science Recap:
Neuroplasticity, habit formation, and metabolic regulation require consistent inputs. Change must be encoded through both mindset and behavior.

Chapter 4: Stop Self-Sabotage Before It Starts

Leadership Insight:
You can't lead others past places where you keep sabotaging yourself. Self-sabotage is not weakness—it's an unhealed

wound operating in secrecy. Awareness is the first leadership skill.

Faith Recap:
Ephesians 4:22–24 calls us to put off the old self and be made new in the attitude of our minds.

Science Recap:
Self-sabotage is a loop triggered by fear, reward-seeking, or subconscious beliefs. Behavioral loops become neurologically ingrained unless consciously interrupted.

Chapter 5: Personality, Patterns & Power...Oh My!

Leadership Insight:
If you don't understand how you're wired, you'll force strategies that don't fit. Great leaders lead themselves first—and personalization is the key to consistency.

Faith Recap:
Proverbs 24:3–4 reminds us that wisdom, understanding, and knowledge build a house. Self-awareness is not self-idolatry—it's spiritual maturity.

Science Recap:
Behavioral styles impact how habits form, how stress is managed, and which environments support or sabotage change. Leadership style must align with health strategy.

Chapter 6: The CEO Reset™

Leadership Insight:
You are the CEO of your health. Energy is a business asset.

You can't make clear decisions if your body is in a constant stress state.

Faith Recap:
God is a God of order (1 Corinthians 14:40). Operating from divine discipline means managing what God gave you—your body, your mind, your influence.

Science Recap:
A regulated nervous system supports executive function, emotional intelligence, and metabolic stability. Burnout and inflammation impair cognition and clarity.

Chapter 7: Make Your Next Move Your Best Move

Leadership Insight:
Every next level requires a new level of self-leadership. You can't wait until you're motivated—you must move with discipline and vision.

Faith Recap:
Proverbs 31:25 reminds us that strength and dignity are our clothing. Trusting God to become who He designed you to be is the foundation of confident leadership.

Science Recap:
Purpose-driven behavior increases dopamine and creates motivation loops. Midlife hormone shifts can be leveraged—not feared—when supported by structure and awareness.

Chapter 8: Divine Discipline

Leadership Insight:
Discipline isn't punishment—it's preparation. It's how leaders build legacy. Without self-governance, your vision becomes vulnerable.

Faith Recap:
Hebrews 12:11 affirms that discipline produces a harvest of righteousness and peace for those who have been trained by it.

Science Recap:
Discipline rewires your brain's reward system. It restores metabolic rhythm, emotional regulation, and long-term resilience.

Chapter 9: Your New Way Forward

Leadership Insight:
Leadership is sustained in daily decisions. What you automate determines what you can scale. The future you're called to lead requires new systems, not just new goals.

Faith Recap:
2 Corinthians 8:11 reminds us to complete the work we started. The pivot isn't finished when you understand it. It's finished when you live it.

Science Recap:
Consistency reinforces neuroplasticity and metabolic stability. Structured routines strengthen identity and reduce mental fatigue.

Your 90-Day Action Plan: Creating The Future You're Called To Lead

"Write the vision and make it plain..."
— **Habakkuk 2:2**

By now, you know this pivot wasn't just about your health. It was about your **habits**, your **identity**, and your **assignment**. This 90-day action plan is not a one-size-fits-all checklist. It's a **leadership protocol** for the most important organization you'll ever run—**you**.

Whether you're leading in the boardroom, at the pulpit, in your home, or through your influence online, you cannot sustain vision on fumes. You need structure. You need strategy. You need stewardship.

This plan is broken into three core phases:

- **Reset** – Strip the noise. Clarify your rhythm.
- **Rebuild** – Lay a sustainable foundation for health and consistency.
- **Reclaim** – Step fully into alignment with your next-level capacity.

You don't have to do this perfectly. You just have to do it *on purpose*.

Let this be your practical guide to move from **knowing what to do** to **becoming the woman who actually does it**.

Print it. Post it. Pray through it.
Then—**walk it out.**

Because this time, you're not just pivoting.
You're rising—with clarity, confidence, and conviction.

This is your blueprint. No perfection required—just commitment. Let's get to work.

MONTH 1: RESET

Focus: Remove noise, restore rhythm

- Establish a non-negotiable morning routine (Scripture, protein, prayer, stillness)
- Remove energy-draining foods (sugar, soda, ultra-processed snacks)
- Walk 20–30 minutes daily—no phone, just presence
- Begin food awareness (track *patterns*, not calories)
- Sleep: in bed before 10:30 p.m., no screens 30 minutes prior

MONTH 2: REBUILD

Focus: Strengthen structure, rewire habits

- Add strength training 2–3x/week (short, intentional sessions)
- Plan your meals 24 hours ahead—keep it simple, balanced, fuel-based
- Implement a Sunday prep routine: food, calendar, mental reset
- Reinforce identity with daily declarations
- Prioritize one act of rest per day (non-productive rest)

MONTH 3: RECLAIM

Focus: Lead yourself like you lead others

- Protect your boundaries (start with one area: food, time, social media)
- Share your story—privately or publicly—to release shame
- Commit to an overflow strategy: what fills you physically, emotionally, spiritually?
- Choose one leadership decision each week that flows from your wellness (not your worry)
- Declare: "This is my new normal. I lead from wholeness."

FINAL THOUGHTS

You did the hard part. You told yourself the truth. You stopped settling for survival. And I am so proud of you. This book alone won't change your life. But the woman you're becoming as you live it out? She will.

She'll make better decisions. She'll take up space with peace. She'll walk in rooms already knowing who she is. She won't lead from burnout. She'll lead from conviction.

And that's why this book isn't about weight loss, workouts, meal plans. It's a leadership manual for your next level.

Welcome to it.

ABOUT THE AUTHOR

Yolanda Moore is a two-time WNBA Champion, award-winning college basketball coach, former executive at Nike and Amazon, and now a nationally recognized Health & Mindset Strategist for women in leadership.

She knows what it means to win on paper—and still feel like you're losing yourself in the process.

A teen mom who went on to earn her degrees while raising two daughters, surviving three knee surgeries, grieving the loss of both parents, and making a professional basketball team just four months postpartum, Yolanda built her life on perseverance. But it wasn't until she faced the emotional wreckage of job loss, career disappointments, depression, and chronic health issues that she finally surrendered—and pivoted.

After losing more than 80 pounds in 8 months, reversing her pre-diabetes and high blood pressure, and releasing the shame that came with chasing success while silently suffering, Yolanda birthed *Pivot Your Way to Health*—not just a brand, but a movement.

Her coaching frameworks integrate neuroscience, biblical truth, and real-world systems to help women stop self-sabotaging and lead from clarity—not chaos. She helps executives, entrepreneurs, and high-achieving women reclaim their energy, authority, and confidence by stewarding their health with purpose.

Yolanda is the founder of **Pivot to Health Enterprises, LLC**, a faith-rooted coaching and wellness company that equips women over 40 to transform their health and elevate their leadership.

She is a mother, grandmother, author, keynote speaker, and vessel for women who are ready to rise.

MEDIA, SPEAKING, & PARTNERSHIPS

Book Yolanda Moore for Your Next Event, Podcast, or Platform

Yolanda is a transformational speaker and thought leader who brings **bold truth, practical strategy, and spiritual power** to every room she enters. She speaks with the authority of someone who's lived what she teaches—and she isn't afraid to tell the truth that sets women free.

From boardrooms and church pulpits to summits, panels, and podcasts—Yolanda brings an unforgettable voice to conversations about:

- Leading while healing
- Health as a spiritual strategy for high-level leadership
- How faith, science, and systems intersect to create sustainable transformation
- Weight loss, wellness, and the Black woman's journey through midlife
- Self-sabotage, burnout recovery, and high-achiever health resets
- Pivoting after personal and professional collapse

Signature Keynote Topics Include:

- *"Pivot Your Way to Health to Reclaim Your Power, Restore Your Confidence, and Lead with Purpose"*
- *"Leverage: 10 Questions to Empower You to Make Your Next Move Your Best Move"*
- *"God Doesn't Want You Sick: How to Reclaim Your Authority Through Stewardship"*
- *You Will Win If You Don't Quit: Developing the Mindset, Beliefs, and Actions of a Champion*

To connect with Yolanda, book an interview, or inquire about speaking:

Visit: www.yolandamoore.com
Email: yolanda@yolandamoore.com
Follow: @iamyolandamoore across all social platforms

Let's shift the culture of success—and show women that **wholeness is the real win.**

www.ingramcontent.com/pod-product-compliance
Lightning Source LLC
Chambersburg PA
CBHW020545030426
42337CB00013B/980